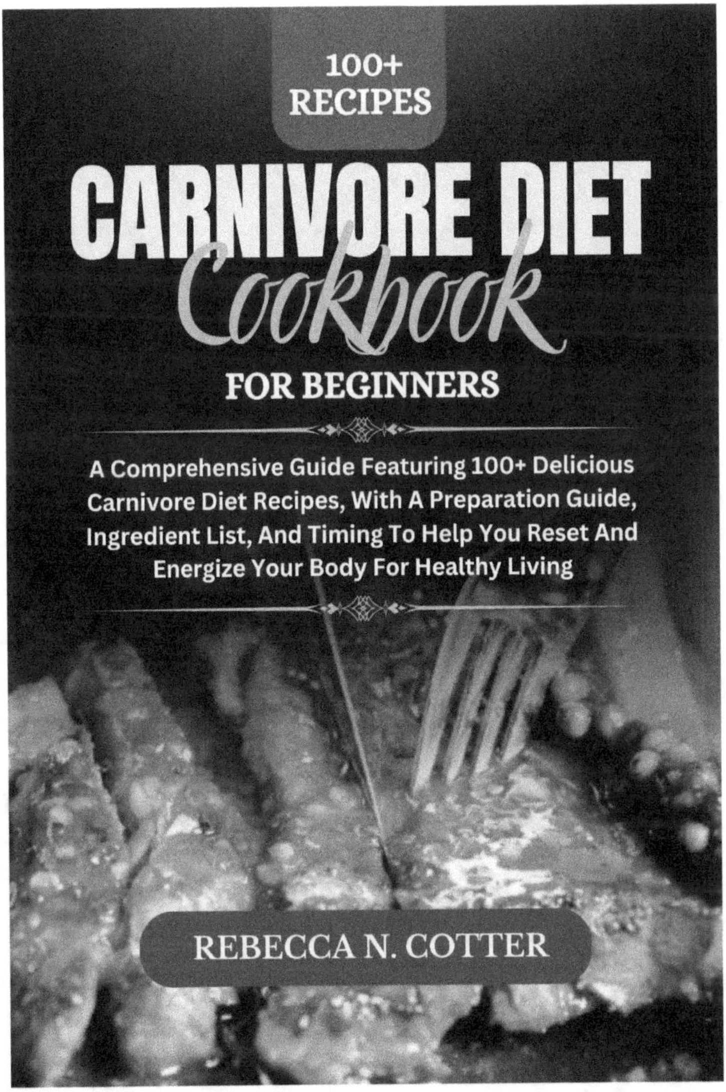

100+
RECIPES

CARNIVORE DIET
Cookbook
FOR BEGINNERS

A Comprehensive Guide Featuring 100+ Delicious
Carnivore Diet Recipes, With A Preparation Guide,
Ingredient List, And Timing To Help You Reset And
Energize Your Body For Healthy Living

REBECCA N. COTTER

CARNIVORE DIET COOKBOOK FOR BEGINNERS:

A Comprehensive Guide Featuring 100+ Delicious Carnivore Diet Recipes, With A Preparation Guide, Ingredient List, And Timing To Help You Reset And Energize Your Body For Healthy Living

Rebecca N. Cotter

Copyright

Disclaimer:

The main objective of this book is to provide comprehensive information on the Carnivore Diet in the form of a cookbook, especially for beginners. However, the information provided is not intended to replace expert medical advice, diagnosis, or treatment. It is recommended to always consult a doctor or other licensed healthcare professional if you have any questions or concerns regarding a medical condition.

Please note that this book does not serve as a customized medical plan, but rather a guide. As every individual's nutritional needs vary, it is always advisable to discuss your dietary changes with a healthcare provider before making any significant adjustments.

Dedication

I dedicate this book to my beloved husband and to all the individuals out there who are devoted to the carnivore diet and aspire to explore its advantages and improve their lives.

Table Of Content

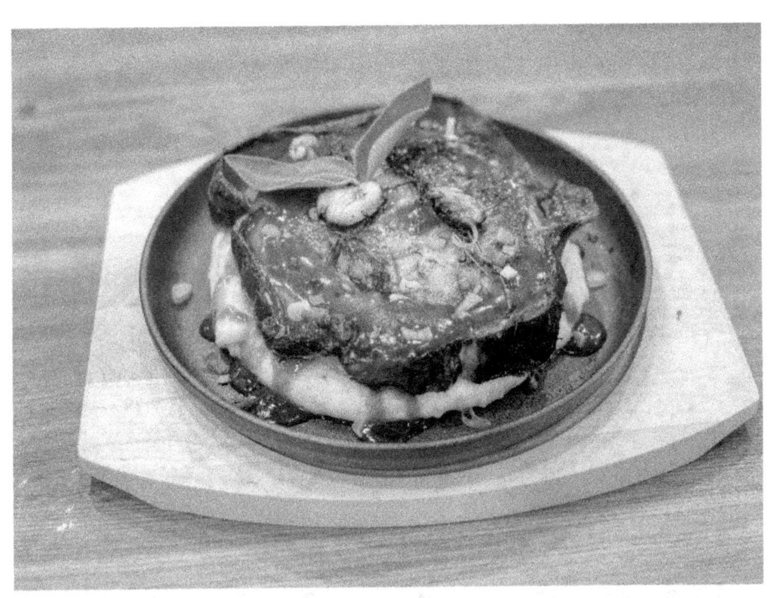

Introduction

Why This Book?

Have you ever felt like your body is trying to tell you something? Perhaps it's the sluggishness you feel after a big meal or the persistent cravings that are hard to resist. If you can relate, you're not alone. I've been there too, trying to navigate the confusing maze of fad diets and conflicting dietary recommendations. That's why I wrote "Carnivore Diet Cookbook for Beginners." It's not just another cookbook, but a guide to restoring your energy and improving your relationship with food. Let me explain why this book can be a life-changing resource on your journey to optimal health and well-being.

> ➤ *Adopting a Carnivorous Lifestyle:*

Choosing a carnivorous diet can be challenging, but it's also a courageous decision. As someone who has experienced the life-changing benefits of this way of eating, I wanted to create a tool that helps newcomers to the lifestyle adjust easily and enjoyably. "Carnivore Diet Cookbook for Beginners" is your guide to embracing a carnivorous diet with comfort and confidence.

> *Not Just Recipes:*

This book features over 100+ delicious recipes that have been carefully crafted to tantalize your taste buds while nourishing your body. But "Carnivore Diet Cookbook for Beginners" is more than just a recipe book. It's a comprehensive handbook that covers everything from scheduling and ingredient selection to meal planning and preparation. Whether you're new to meat-eating or a seasoned carnivore, this book has something for everyone on their path to optimal health.

Starting a new eating plan can be daunting, but it doesn't have to be. That's why I've included practical advice and techniques throughout the book to make it easier for you to adopt a carnivorous lifestyle. These tips range from time-saving meal prep methods to kitchen basics and are designed to help you succeed on your carnivorous journey.

➤ *Encouraging You to Take Control:*

The ultimate goal of "The Carnivore Diet Cookbook for Beginners" is to empower you to take control of your health and well-being. This book gives you the information, resources, and techniques you need to thrive on a carnivorous diet. Say goodbye to restrictive diets and hello to a lifestyle that fuels your spirit and nurtures your body.

➤ *Transformative Benefits:*

The carnivore diet is about harnessing the transformative power of good nutrition, not just weight loss or surface-level improvements. By fueling your body with high-quality nutrients, you'll experience a renewed sense of vitality and well-being. The benefits of the carnivorous diet extend beyond the dinner table, including increased energy and improved mental clarity.

"Carnivore Diet Cookbook for Beginners" is more than just a recipe book. It's your ticket to a happier, healthier life. Whether you're looking to reset your health, invigorate your body, or simply try a new way of eating, this book has everything you need to succeed on your carnivore journey. So why wait? Take a deep breath, look around, and start on the path to a happier, healthier version of yourself.

Who Should Follow the Carnivore Diet?

Are you wondering whether the carnivore diet is right for you? Look no further! This lifestyle is adaptable and perfect for a broad range of individuals seeking a holistic approach to wellness. That's what makes it so magnificent. As the author of "Carnivore Diet Cookbook for Beginners," I firmly believe that for those who can relate to its principles, the carnivore diet can be a life-altering experience.

This cookbook is designed for people who are curious and enjoy exploring new options and taking unconventional paths. If you're dedicated to improving your health, the carnivore diet has the potential to be incredibly beneficial. This book provides the resources and recipes to support your health-conscious way of living. If you're feeling lethargic, dealing with recurrent cravings, or just need a reset, the carnivore diet may be the solution. This book will guide you through the process of detoxifying and revitalizing your body with nutrient-dense, carnivorous food. It's created for those seeking a reset.

The advantages of a carnivorous diet go beyond physical health to include improved concentration and mental clarity. If you're looking to enhance your cognitive function and mental clarity, this book provides a comprehensive strategy to support your mental health objectives. Fitness enthusiasts seeking a nutritional plan that fits into their busy lifestyle can find the missing piece in the carnivore diet. The recipes in this book are designed to meet the needs of fitness enthusiasts and promote muscle health and recovery. They are packed with protein and essential nutrients.

If you've been struggling with dietary allergies and want an eating plan that works for your body's requirements, the carnivore diet may be worth considering. This lifestyle emphasizes whole foods and reduces potential allergens and irritants, making it a viable option for people with specific dietary concerns. "Carnivore Diet Cookbook for Beginners" is a tailored guidebook thoughtfully designed to meet the diverse needs and goals of people from all backgrounds who are open to embracing a carnivorous lifestyle for self-discovery and wellness. If the concepts of the carnivorous diet resonate with you, pick up this book and begin your journey toward transformation with confidence.

Chapter 1

CARNIVORE DIET BASICS

Understanding The Carnivore Diet

As the author of "Carnivore Diet Cookbook for Beginners," I want to guide you through the life-changing experience of starting a carnivorous diet. It involves a deep understanding and nourishment of your body at a unique and profound level. In this book, I will take you on a thorough tour of this way of life, covering its main tenets, the science behind them, and the essential elements that combine to create a comprehensive approach to health.

> ➤*Here Are The Key Principles Of The Carnivore Diet:*

1. Animal-based nutrition is the cornerstone of the carnivore diet. Meats take center stage because they are a rich source of vital nutrients that are consistent with the evolutionary history of human dietary patterns. These include beef, poultry, fish, and organ meats.

2. The diet emphasizes nutrient-dense foods. This means eating foods that are

high in nutrients rather than just consuming calories. Organ meats are particularly noteworthy because they contain concentrated amounts of vitamins, minerals, and other nutrients that are vital to general health.

3. The carnivorous diet involves decreasing or completely eliminating plant-based foods. This is to reduce allergens, anti-nutrients, and potential irritants in specific plants to create a diet that is easy on the digestive tract.

4. Quality is important. Choosing meat from grass-fed, pasture-raised, and wild-caught animals guarantees that the meat you eat is not only higher in

nutrients than other types of meat but also free of any possible contaminants that may be present in animals raised conventionally.

> ➤ *Here Is The Empirical Evidence That Supports The Carnivore Diet:*

1. The diet is based on our evolutionary history and how our ancestors survived on diets high in animal products. Animal products are a natural and bioavailable source of nutrition because the human digestive system has evolved to effectively extract nutrients from them.

2. High nutrient bioavailability—the body's ability to readily absorb and use the nutrients—is a characteristic of animal-based sources. By doing this, you can maximize the benefits of each bite and promote optimal body functions.

3. Protein is essential because it acts as a fundamental building block by supplying the necessary amino acids needed for immunological response, tissue repair, and the production of important hormones and enzymes.

4. The carnivore diet celebrates the healthy fats found in animal products, in contrast to conventional fatphobia. These fats, which include both saturated and

monounsaturated fats, support healthy brain function, hormone regulation, and long-term energy levels.

The carnivore diet is made up of vital elements that combine to form a comprehensive strategy for overall health:

1. A varied nutrient profile is ensured by embracing a range of meats. Every type of meat, including poultry, fatty fish, and red meats like beef and lamb, has specific nutritional advantages of its own.

2. Organ meats are particularly rich in nutrients. Vital minerals like iron and zinc, as well as vitamins A, B, D, E, and K, are abundant in the liver, heart, and kidney.

You can increase the variety of nutrients in your diet by including organ meats.

3. Animal-based healthy fats are an essential ingredient. Tallow, lard, and fatty meat cuts offer a steady energy source and improve general health.

4. Drinking enough water is essential to support healthy digestion and general body functions, although water is naturally found in meat.

As a beginner, you should comprehend the basics of the carnivore diet, recognize the important elements that support its holistic approach, and appreciate the science behind its tenets. Allow the individualized wisdom and thorough knowledge found in "Carnivore Diet Cookbook for Beginners" to lead you on this life-changing journey toward a well-fed, vibrant, and energetic existence.

> *Difference Between A Plant-based Diets And Carnivore Diet .*

1. Plant-Based Diet:

A plant-based diet focuses on eating foods that are derived from plants, such as grains, legumes, nuts, seeds, fruits, and vegetables. This way of eating emphasizes the variety of plant-based foods while reducing or eliminating animal products completely. Advocates of a plant-based diet typically point to health, environmental, and ethical grounds for their dietary decisions, promoting a diet high in fiber, antioxidants, and phytonutrients, all of which are abundant in plant-based foods. With a plant-based diet, the emphasis is on encouraging sustainability, minimizing the impact on the environment, and enhancing general wellbeing.

2. Carnivore Diet:

The carnivore diet advocates for using foods derived from animals as the main source of nutrition. This kind of eating emphasizes eating as much meat, fish, eggs, and other animal products as possible, and consuming very little or no plant-based food. The evolutionary biology-inspired carnivore diet places a strong emphasis on the nutrient density and bioavailability of animal products. Dieters who follow the carnivore diet frequently attribute their dietary choices to improvements in their general health, energy levels, and mental clarity. Simplifying food choices, maximizing nutrient intake, and adopting a diet that is in line with our evolutionary past as carnivorous organisms are the main goals.

> *Benefits of Carnivore Diet:*

Starting a carnivore diet is an invitation to experience a wave of life-changing advantages that reverberate throughout your entire being, rather than just a change in eating habits. Allow me to lead you on a personalized journey to discover the incomparable advantages that this way of life can offer.

1. Increase in Vitality and Energy:
The increase in energy levels is one of the most significant advantages of the carnivore diet. You supply a consistent and effective source of energy for your body when you feed it nutrient-dense animal foods. Many report feeling renewable energetic, no longer experiencing the energy slumps brought on by processed

carbohydrates and feeling consistent, natural energy all day long.

2. Emotional Focus and Clarity:
Benefits of the carnivore diet go beyond physical health to include improved mental and cognitive performance. Increased focus, better concentration, and mental acuity are frequently reported by followers. When you provide your brain with the vital nutrients that are present in animal products, you set yourself up for success in both physical and cognitive domains.

3. Controlling Body Weight and Composition:

The carnivore diet can be a game-changer for people looking for a revolutionary approach to weight management. People frequently see improvements in their body composition, including fat loss and an increase in lean muscle mass, by cutting out processed foods and concentrating on nutrient-dense animal sources. It is also simpler to control calorie intake with this simple diet.

4. Digestive Harmony and Gut Health:
Despite worries about how it may affect digestion, many people discover that a carnivorous diet actually improves gut health and digestive balance. Followers frequently report relief from gastrointestinal problems, decreased

bloating, and an overall more comfortable experience by reducing or eliminating specific plant-based irritants.

5. Equilibrium Blood Sugar Levels:
Blood sugar levels are kept in check by the carnivore diet's emphasis on protein and good fats. Followers frequently report more consistent energy levels and fewer cravings when they consume fewer refined carbohydrates and sugars. This feature is especially helpful for people who want to control or avoid conditions that are associated with blood sugar swings.

6. Increased Sports Efficiency:
Athletic performance often improves for fitness enthusiasts who adopt a

carnivorous lifestyle. Superior proteins, necessary fats, and an ideal nutrient intake promote muscle repair, recuperation, and general physical stamina. The carnivore diet can be a helpful ally in achieving your performance objectives, regardless of whether you're an athlete or just someone who exercises frequently.

7. Easier Nutritional Decisions:

The carnivore diet offers simplicity in an age of confusing dietary fads and contradictory nutritional advice. The simple eating philosophy, which emphasizes whole, unprocessed animal foods, is frequently appreciated by adherents. This ease of use not only facilitates meal preparation but also encourages a more intuitive approach to body nourishment and a closer relationship with food.

Taking up the carnivore diet is more than just a food experiment; it's an investigation of maximum health, energy, and a balance between body and diet. May the advantages that you experience along this journey of transformation align specifically with your health objectives and desires.

➤ *How Often Should You Eat On The Carnivore Diet?*

The Carnivore Diet is flexible, allowing you to customize how often you eat to suit your preferences and lifestyle. Unlike strict eating plans, the Carnivore Diet lets you eat intuitively, following your body's signals. Some people thrive on two or three meals per day, while others adopt intermittent fasting, which involves extended intervals between meals to maximize fat burning and metabolic flexibility.

The key is to find a rhythm that maintains your energy levels and meets your body's needs. Pay attention to cues related to hunger and satiety and prioritize nutrient-dense animal foods, whether you prefer regular meals or intermittent fasting. Remember that the Carnivore Diet is all about feeding your body in a way that suits your physiology, not following rigid guidelines. To create a sustainable and unique approach to the carnivore lifestyle, let your hunger and energy levels dictate how often you eat.

> ➤ *What Are The Side Effects Of Starting A Carnivorous Diet?*

Starting a carnivore diet can be a life-changing experience, but like any lifestyle change, it may require some initial adjustments. These transient symptoms are often referred to as the "keto flu" or "carnivore flu," and they frequently signify your body adjusting to a new metabolic state. During the initial shift, some people may experience headaches, fatigue, or irritability as their body adjusts to using fat instead of carbs as its primary energy source. This stage is usually transient and can be lessened by drinking plenty of water, making sure you're getting enough electrolytes, and giving your body time to adjust.

Additionally, as the gut adjusts to a diet high in animal products, some people may experience digestive changes, such as changes in bowel habits. During this period of adjustment, maintaining a sufficient intake of fiber and drinking plenty of water can help maintain digestive health. It's critical to approach these possible negative symptoms with self-compassion and patience. Your body is going through a metamorphosis, and the short-term difficulties are frequently followed by long-term gains from a carnivorous diet.

> ➤ *How To Overcome Potentially Negative Symptoms*

When transitioning to a carnivorous diet, it's important to be self-aware, patient, and take proactive steps to aid your body's adaptation process to minimize any possible side effects.

1. Drink plenty of water: Staying hydrated is essential for optimal function and assisting your body's detoxification processes. To stay hydrated and eliminate toxins from your body, try to drink a lot of water throughout the day.

2. Balance your electrolytes: Make sure you're rehydrating electrolytes, like potassium, sodium, and magnesium, particularly in the beginning stages of adjustment. In order to maintain proper hydration and avoid imbalances, think about including foods or supplements high in electrolytes in your diet.

3. Gradual Transition: If your symptoms are severe, gradually reducing your

carbohydrate intake can facilitate the transition process and lessen the shock to your system.

4. Monitor your nutrient intake: To meet your body's needs, make sure you're getting a variety of foods derived from animals and pay attention to the nutrients you're consuming. Nutrient-dense seafood and organ meats can supply vital vitamins and minerals to promote general health.

5. Listen to your body: Above all, pay attention to the signals your body gives you and respect your unique needs. Consider changing your strategy if specific foods or eating habits make your

symptoms worse. By emphasizing electrolyte balance, hydration, nutrient intake, gradual transition, and self-awareness, you can avoid unpleasant side effects and make a smooth transition to the carnivore diet.

Chapter 2

MEAT GUIDE SELECTION

What are the best meat options for a carnivorous diet? Although any type of meat is acceptable except for substitutes like Beyond Meat, some cuts and varieties are better than others.

Here are our top picks for meat choices on a carnivorous diet, starting with the classic choice for carnivores: red meats.

1. Red Meats: Lamb, Pork, and Beef

Research shows that animal-derived cholesterol is not intrinsically harmful, although red meat is frequently criticized for its high cholesterol content. Good cholesterol levels may even be encouraged by natural fats. For additional information, see our article on the carnivore diet and cholesterol. Meanwhile, the following are the best meat options for a carnivorous diet:

- Beef: Packed with vital nutrients like zinc, iron, and vitamin B12, this protein source is highly nutritious. It also provides high-quality protein and saturated fats that are essential for cellular health and energy production. Grass-fed beef has higher concentrations of antioxidants and omega-3 fatty acids.

- Lamb: This nutrient-rich meat is frequently underappreciated. It is a good source of protein, rich in vitamins B12 and B3, and loaded with minerals like zinc and selenium. Its higher fat content—especially in those raised on grass—provides essential fatty acids.

- Pork: A carnivore's diet can benefit greatly from the inclusion of pork, especially fatty cuts. Rich in B vitamins, especially B1 (thiamine), which is ironically important for the metabolism of carbohydrates given the low-carb nature of the diet. Pork also provides high-quality protein and bioavailable heme iron.

2. Poultry: Duck, Turkey, and Chicken
Although the carnivore diet doesn't demonize fat, some people choose leaner options to help with their weight loss efforts. Carnivores can find poultry to be a great alternative to T-bone steaks when they're looking for something lighter.

- Chicken: Known for being versatile, chicken provides a lean protein source that is lower in fat than red meats. It provides vital nutrients such as selenium and niacin, and it is advantageous for individuals watching their calorie intake.

- Turkey: Another excellent source of protein, turkey is similar to chicken but frequently leaner. It has high levels of B vitamins, which are essential for generating energy, and is a good source of selenium.

- Duck: Flavored and rich in nutrients, a duck has a unique nutritional makeup. Compared to chicken or turkey, it has a higher fat content. It is also a great source of iron, B vitamins, and niacin, which supports healthy skin and metabolism.

3. Marine Delight: Fish and Shellfish

Prime meat options for a carnivore diet aren't limited to land, despite popular belief. For those looking for lighter yet nutrient-dense options, seafood provides an additional option. The range of recipes goes beyond salmon grilled to include:

- Fish: Packed with omega-3 fatty acids, fish—especially oily types like salmon, mackerel, and sardines—are essential for cardiovascular and cognitive health. It provides high-quality protein and important vitamins, like B12 and D, which are frequently lacking in a diet high in meat.

- Shellfish: Clams, mussels, and oysters stand out as nutrient-dense powerhouses. Packed with zinc and vitamin B12, they are essential for supporting healthy metabolism and the immune system. Particularly oysters have a higher zinc content per serving than other foods, which is important for immune system and metabolic health.

4. Organ Meats: Kidney, Heart, and Liver

Diversity in the carnivore diet is important for ensuring a wide range of nutrients, not just for taste. This is where organ meats come in.

These meats take some getting used to, but they eventually become more flavorful. You can also incorporate them into recipes for carnivore diets to make them more palatable; as time goes on, you should find yourself craving them more and more. Here are the essentials:

- Liver: Known as the multivitamin of nature, liver has a remarkable nutrient density. Rich in vitamin A, which is essential for eyesight, and brimming with iron and B vitamins, especially B12, it is a foundational food.

- Kidney: Rich in B12 and riboflavin (B2), kidneys offer a unique nutritional profile full of selenium, iron, and B vitamins.

- Heart: Packed full of muscle, the heart is a rich source of CoQ10, a nutrient vital to cardiovascular health and energy production. It is also an excellent source of iron, zinc, and B vitamins.

> *Essential Tools for Carnivore Cooking*

When starting your carnivore diet, make sure your kitchen has everything you need to make preparation simple. These accessories help your carnivorous culinary journey succeed in addition to making cooking easier.

1. Cooking Utensils: A good set of cooking utensils, such as tongs, spatulas, and a sharp knife, guarantees that meat is handled effectively both during preparation and cooking.

2. Slow-Cooker/Crock Pot: A slow cooker is perfect for slow-cooking meats to perfection because it can intensify flavors, tenderize tough cuts, and produce results that melt in your mouth.

3. Meat Thermometer: Use a meat thermometer to make sure your meat is safe to eat and has reached the right

doneness. For perfectly cooked meals, you can monitor internal temperatures with the aid of this tool.

4. Roasting Pan with Rack Insert: When roasting large cuts of meat, a roasting pan with a rack insert is a necessity. By raising the meat, the rack promotes even cooking and ideal air circulation.

5. Dutch Oven: A Dutch oven is a multipurpose kitchen tool that works well for stewing, braising, and slow-cooking meats. Its substantial walls evenly distribute heat for outstanding outcomes.

6. Cast Iron Skillet: For searing and frying meat, a cast iron skillet works great

because it forms a flavorful crust and retains juices. It is a long-lasting addition to your carnivorous kitchen because of its durability.

7. Grill Pan or Grill: Use an outdoor grill or a stovetop grill pan to savor the flavor of grilled meat. Your carnivorous dishes take on a delightful smokiness from the grill, which also improves the taste and texture.

8. Meat Tenderizer: A meat tenderizer is ideal for removing the fibers from more densely cut meat, guaranteeing that your carnivorous meals are not only flavorful but also incredibly tender.

9. Cutting Board Set: Cross-contamination can be avoided by using a set of sturdy cutting boards specifically meant for meat preparation. To ensure hygienic conditions in your carnivorous kitchen, use distinct boards for different types of meat.

10. Food Storage Containers: Meat prep, leftovers, and carnivorous meals prepared in bulk should be kept in airtight storage containers. This guarantees freshness and facilitates meal planning.

If you stock your kitchen with these necessities, you'll be ready to tackle the carnivore diet. These products help you enjoy and succeed in your carnivorous lifestyle in addition to making cooking

easier.

Chapter 3

CHOLESTEROL AND CARNIVORE

How Does It Affect Cholesterol Levels?

The word "cholesterol" can cause anxiety, especially in this day and age when heart disease is so common. Discussions concerning cholesterol levels have become a regular occurrence, with people looking for information to better comprehend the consequences. But in all the anxiety, a diet trend known as the carnivore diet has surfaced, promising alleged health benefits.

The carnivore diet deviates from traditional dietary guidelines by emphasizing meat-centric meals with little to no plant-based content. However, a lot of people have mentioned significant health gains while on this regimen, which has raised questions about its possible advantages. However, one question remains unanswered, clouding the apparent benefits of this dietary strategy: Does the carnivore diet raise or lower cholesterol?

You're in the right place if you've been wondering about the precise connection between cholesterol and the carnivore diet. Concerning the carnivore diet, this extensive guide seeks to shed light on the subject of cholesterol. We'll go into detail about how the carnivore diet affects cholesterol levels so you can make an informed decision about your health. Let's quickly review the carnivore diet and cholesterol before we go any further. Because of the complex interactions between diet and cholesterol, it is important to have a basic understanding of each. Let's get familiar with these basic ideas before delving deeper into this relationship.

➤ *Understanding Cholesterol: Hdl vs. Ldl*

Essential roles for cholesterol include the synthesis of vitamin D, the production of hormones, and support for the digestive system. High cholesterol has long been associated with negative health effects. But not every cholesterol is made equally. There are two main kinds of lipoproteins: LDL (low-density lipoprotein) and HDL (high-density lipoprotein), both of which are important.

Known as "bad" cholesterol, low-density lipoprotein (LDL) carries cholesterol from the liver to cells that need it. In comparison to HDL, excessive levels of LDL cholesterol can build up on arterial walls, causing plaque to form, artery narrowing, and an increased risk of heart disease and stroke. HDL cholesterol, on the other hand, is considered "good" cholesterol since it helps move cholesterol from cells back to the liver where it is eliminated from the body. Lower risks of heart disease and stroke are linked to high levels of HDL cholesterol.

Therefore, rather than concentrating only on lowering total cholesterol levels, overall health must maintain a balance between LDL and HDL cholesterol. There is no denying the link between cholesterol and a carnivorous diet. The specifics of this relationship are still up for discussion, though. Does a carnivorous diet raise cholesterol or does it help those who already have high cholesterol? Let's look at both viewpoints.

➤ *Does A Carnivorous Diet Raise Your Cholesterol Levels?*

It's not easy to answer whether a carnivorous diet increases cholesterol. A lot of people who start a carnivorous diet initially notice a rise in their cholesterol. The main cause of this phenomenon is the consumption of meat's high saturated fat content, which causes the liver to produce more cholesterol.

But it's important to understand that cholesterol isn't always bad for you. As was previously mentioned, cholesterol is essential to the body. As a result, striking a balance between LDL and HDL cholesterol should be the main goal. Furthermore, a comprehensive evaluation of health is essential. Even though some people may experience increases in cholesterol, other health markers like improved blood sugar control, decreased inflammation, and weight loss may also show improvements, which could lessen the risks.

> *Can Cholesterol Be Reduced By A Carnivorous Diet?*

On the other hand, might a carnivorous diet eventually lower cholesterol? It's interesting to note that an extended carnivore diet may help maintain a better cholesterol profile, according to some research and anecdotal evidence. Considering the high saturated fat content of the diet, how does this seemingly contradictory outcome occur?

Eliminating carbs, especially refined sugars and grains, is probably a key component. These food items have the potential to cause insulin resistance and inflammation, two major causes of elevated cholesterol. Some people may have lower LDL and higher HDL cholesterol after removing these variables, which would promote a better overall balance.

Furthermore, the high protein content of the carnivore diet may aid in weight loss, which is frequently linked to lower cholesterol levels. Individual reactions to the carnivore diet, however, differ greatly. Moreover, it is imperative to recognize the paucity of research on the effects of the carnivore diet on cholesterol, which calls for additional study before any firm conclusions can be drawn.

➢ *Should High Cholesterol On A Carnivore Diet Be Considered Dangerous?*

Considering the contradictory results regarding cholesterol, one might reasonably wonder if concerns about high cholesterol on a carnivorous diet are justified.

The bottom line is that, although it's important to monitor any changes in cholesterol levels when implementing a carnivorous diet, you might not need to act immediately on this. Recall that cholesterol is a necessary substance that the body needs and is not intrinsically dangerous. As an alternative, concentrate on reaching a healthy balance between LDL and HDL cholesterol, general health, and personal dietary responses.

Moreover, there are a lot of health advantages to the carnivore diet, such as decreased inflammation, better blood sugar regulation, and weight loss, which may outweigh worries about cholesterol. It's also critical to understand that dietary decisions are only one part of managing cholesterol and maintaining general heart health. Significant influences on cholesterol levels are also exerted by factors like stress levels, physical activity, alcohol and tobacco use, genetic predispositions, and stress levels.

Our suggestion? As you begin your dietary journey, keep an eye on your cholesterol levels and monitor any changes with professional guidance. Routine assessments can reveal worrying trends, in which case changes can be made to ensure peace of mind while actively pursuing better physical and mental well-being. Additionally, if you still have concerns about high cholesterol while following the carnivore diet, keep reading for tips on controlling cholesterol levels.

➤ *Ways to Reduce Cholesterol on a Carnivorous Diet*

It's not always the case that switching to a carnivorous diet means giving up control over cholesterol. People can properly control their cholesterol levels and enjoy the advantages of a carnivorous diet by making thoughtful decisions and tactical tweaks. Think about putting these pointers into practice:

1. Make Lean Cuts a Priority: Choose leaner meat cuts to lower your intake of saturated fat and support a healthier cholesterol profile.

2. Include Seafood: To strengthen heart health, include seafood high in omega-3 fatty acids, such as salmon and mackerel.

Select Leaner Meat Options

Different types of meat have different amounts of fat and cholesterol. Choosing leaner meats will help reduce your intake of saturated fat, which will help control your cholesterol. Think about alternatives like turkey, lean ground beef, or skinless chicken breast. Although meat is the main component of the carnivore diet, every meal doesn't need to include a thick steak.

One of the best ways to get access to lean protein sources is to include fish in your diet. Fish also contains omega-3 fatty acids, which are known to have positive effects on the heart and lower cholesterol. Frequent additions of fatty fish, such as sardines, mackerel, and salmon, can promote cholesterol balance.

- Take Part in Regular Physical Activity

Regular physical activity is one of the most effective ways to protect heart health and control cholesterol. Exercise helps to raise HDL ("good") cholesterol levels while lowering LDL ("bad") cholesterol levels at the same time. Aim to include 75 minutes of vigorous activity or at least 150 minutes of moderate aerobic activity each week, along with strength training activities.

- Make lifestyle modifications

In addition to dietary changes and exercise programs, other aspects of lifestyle also have an impact on cholesterol levels. These include keeping a healthy weight, consuming alcohol in moderation, and quitting smoking. Making stress management a priority is also essential because high stress levels hurt cholesterol profiles.

- Frequent Evaluation of Cholesterol Regular health monitoring is an essential component of any eating plan. Maintain a schedule of regular blood tests and examinations to monitor cholesterol levels. By taking the proactive route, you and your healthcare provider can determine how your body will react to the carnivore diet and adjust the diet as needed.

Chapter 4

PORK & POULTRY RECIPES

Sear Pork Chops

Preparation 5 minutes || Cooking 15
Minutes

This is a simple and quick recipe for pork chops that you can eat for lunch or dinner. The pork chops have a crispy golden crust, a generous amount of succulent fat surrounding the edges, and a juicy inside.

Ingredients

- Four chops of heritage-bred pork

- Salt
- Cooking fat

Cooking tips:

A variety of steaks can be cooked using this method. If unsure, try pan-searing.

Money-saving advice:

Either boneless or bone-in chops work well in this recipe. Choosing chops with bones can both reduce costs and enhance appearance. After removing any leftover meat, you can also toss the leftover bone into your chicken coop.

Guidelines:

1. Season the pork chops with salt.

2. Heat some cooking fat in a cast-iron or stainless-steel skillet.

3. Sear the pork chops for five minutes on each side, or until a crust forms, in a hot pan. To check the temperature, use a meat thermometer. It reads medium-rare at 145°F (65°C). After that, take the chops out of the skillet.

4. While still warm, let the chops rest for at least five minutes before serving.

Pork Tenderloin Wrapped In Bacon
Preparation 20 minutes || Cooking 40 Minutes

Making a sophisticated dinner of pork tenderloin is simple and can be done by anyone. You can have a five-star recipe on your dining table with just ten minutes of prep work and some baking time.

Ingredients :

- A single tablespoon of salt
- A two-pound tenderloin of heritage pork
- A couple of tsp melted pork fat from Heritage

- Eight to ten pieces of uncooked bacon

Cooking Advice:

Make sure there's enough bacon on the tenderloin to completely envelop it. You may need to use more or less bacon, depending on how big the loin pieces are.

Add-ins with flavor:

Step 2: Combine the salt with a dry rub seasoning to add flavor. Use a sugar-free spice blend if you're following a ketogenic diet.

Guidelines:

1. Set the oven temperature to 425°F (218°C).

2. Season the tenderloin on all sides with salt and generously brush it with lard. After that, put it aside.

3. Arrange the bacon on a cutting board. Sandwich the pork between two bacon strips. Starting from one end, pull the bacon slightly angled at a diagonal over the pork. With the remaining slices, repeat the process by crossing the second side over the first. Tuck the ends under the overlapping slices, and if needed, secure them with toothpicks.

4. After wrapping the pork, place it in a baking dish and bake for 20 minutes.

5. After 20 minutes, lower the heat to 300°F (148°C) and continue baking.

6. Once the internal temperature reaches 135°F (57°C), turn on the broiler and continue cooking for five more minutes.

7. After removing the pork from the oven, tent it with foil, and allow it to rest for ten minutes, then slice and serve it hot.

Crusted Mozzarella Sticks With Bacon

Preparation 5 minutes || Cooking 15 Minutes

Enjoy the flavor of warm, melted cheese and crispy, salty bacon when you wrap mozzarella cheese sticks in bacon. This is how to prepare it:

Ingredients :

- Half a pound of mozzarella cheese
- 12 strips of uncured bacon

Guidelines:

1. Slice the cheese into six substantial pieces.

2. Put parchment paper on the rim of a baking sheet. After placing the cheese sticks on the sheet, freeze them for 60 minutes.

3. Set oven temperature to 400°F or 204°C.

4. Using one bacon strip lengthwise and one widthwise, encircle each cheese stick twice.

5. Bake for fifteen minutes. When hot, serve right away.

Quesadilla for Meat Lovers
Preparation 35 minutes || Cooking 15 Minutes

In this recipe, a "quesadilla" pocket is baked with cheese, bacon, and chicken. It's a tasty and enjoyable way to eat a low-fiber, high-protein meal. This is how to prepare it:

Ingredients :

- 20 strips of uncured bacon
- 2 cups cooked chicken, cut into slices or shreds.
- 1/4 cup of organic cheese, shredded

Add-ins for Flavor:

Utilize any leftover chicken from slow-cooked or oven-roasted whole chicken. You could also use pulled pork instead.

Guidelines:

1. Set oven temperature to 400°F, or 204°C.
2. Use parchment paper to line a baking sheet.
3. Pick ten bacon pieces. Place the first five bacon strips next to one another. To create a second woven bacon square, weave the remaining 5 bacon strips into the first layer in the opposite direction.
4. For thirty minutes, bake.
5. Arrange the chicken on top of the bacon, then top with cheese. Place the other woven bacon square on top.

6. Replace the parchment paper on the sheet with a new one after discarding the old one. Put it back in the oven and let it melt the cheese for about five minutes. Cut in half, then warmly serve.

Pulled Pork
Preparation 10 minutes || Cooking 8–12 Hours

Pork cooked slowly is a wonderful complement to any dish. This is how to prepare it:

Ingredients :
- One cup of chicken or bone broth
- One three-pound pork butt
- One tablespoon of salt

Recipe Advice:
Reheat the pork in a skillet over medium-high heat with a spoonful or two

of Heritage Pork Lard. Cook the meat until it is fried and the edges are crisp.

Guidelines:

1. Set the slow cooker to a low heat. Add the pork butt and broth. Add some salt for seasoning.

2. Cook the pork covered for 8 to 12 hours, or until it easily shreds with a fork.

3. Using two forks, separate the pork once it has been transferred to the serving dish.

4. Serve hot, adding butter or your favorite fat if necessary. Keep any leftovers chilled.

Crock-Pot Baby Back Ribs
Preparation 15 minutes || Cooking 3-4 Minutes

Chicken cooked slowly is a tasty and simple dinner. This is how to prepare it:

Ingredients :

- One whole organic free-range chicken
- Two tablespoons of melted butter, Ghee, or cooking fat
- Two tsp of salt

Add-ins for Flavor:

Dress the chicken with aromatic herbs such as parsley, basil, oregano, and rosemary after seasoning it with salt. Take out before serving, or consume if preferred.

Recipe Advice:

Once cooked, remove the chicken from the pot and transfer it to a 9x13 glass or ceramic baking dish. Put under the broiler for 4−5 minutes, or until the skin is crispy and golden brown. When serving, remove from heat and let sit for five to ten minutes.

Guidelines:

1. In the slow cooker, put the chicken. Apply ghee or butter all over it. Add some salt for seasoning.

2. Cook on low for 6 to 8 hours with a cover on. Warm up the food. Cook the chicken for a variety of times, depending on its size

and the pot, until the internal temperature reaches 165°F (75°C).

Whole Chicken Roasted In The Oven
Preparation 5 minutes || Cooking 1 hour

Roasting a whole chicken should be a skill for every recent high school graduate. It's a quick and practical method for cooking a lot of meat. There are numerous ways to use chicken that has been sliced, cubed, or shredded.

Ingredients

- A whole, five-pound organic, free-range chicken
- 1/4 cup of cooking fat, such as butter or duck fat
- A single tablespoon of salt

Guidelines

1. Set the oven temperature to 425°F (218°C).

2. After rubbing the cooking fat all over the chicken, season it with salt.

3. Roast the chicken in the oven until the internal temperature reaches 165°F (74°C), placing it in a baking dish. When it's done, the skin should be crispy and golden, taking about an hour.

4. Ten minutes should pass before slicing and serving the chicken.

Whole Chicken Bleu Cooked Slowly
Preparation 5 minutes || Cooking 6-8 hours

You can make a chicken dinner with this recipe in the morning and serve it in the late afternoon or early evening. All you have to do is prepare your slow cooker. You can use a range of salts, including smoked salt, black lava salt, and various mineral salts, to improve the flavor of the final dish.

Ingredients

- One whole, organic chicken raised outdoors

- Two tablespoons of ghee, melted
  butter, or cooking fat
- Two salt teaspoons

After seasoning the chicken with salt, sprinkle it with aromatic herbs like basil, parsley, oregano, and rosemary to add even more flavor. If desired, remove the herbs before serving or eating.

Cooking advice:

- After the chicken is done, take it out of the slow cooker and place it in a 9 x 13 baking dish made of glass or ceramic.
- Broil it for four to five minutes, or until the skin is golden brown and crispy.

- Allow it to rest for five to ten minutes before serving.

Guidelines

1. Add the chicken to the slow cooker, completely cover it with cooking fat, butter, or ghee, and season with salt.

2. Place a lid on it and cook on low for a duration of 6 to 8 hours.

3. Reheat the chicken to serve it. The size of the pot and the chicken will affect how long they take to cook. Prior to serving, ensure that the leg's internal temperature reaches 165°F or 75°C.

Chicken Cordon With Four Cheeses
Preparation 15 minutes || Cooking 50 minutes

Four distinct cheeses melt perfectly inside plump, high-protein chicken breasts. The flavor is intense. Serve this gourmet-style dinner to your close friends, family, and any lucky houseguests.

Ingredients :

- 1/4 cup of organic Gruyère cheese, shredded
- Half a cup of organic Swiss cheese, shredded
- One-third cup of organic Raclette cheese, shredded

- Two large, butterflied, boneless, and free-range chicken breasts that have been thinly pounded
- One tablespoon of butter made from grass
- 1/2 cup of organic Parmesan cheese, finely grated
- One teaspoon of salt

Guidelines:

1. Set the oven's temperature to 175°C, or 350°F.

2. Use parchment paper to line a baking sheet.

3. In a bowl, combine the shredded cheeses.

4. After flattening the chicken breasts, divide the cheese mixture in half. To

enclose the cheese, place one half inside each chicken breast and fold.

5. Brush each chicken breast with butter, then top with salt and Parmesan cheese.

6. When the internal temperature of the chicken reaches 165°F (or 75°C), bake it for 50 minutes on the prepared baking sheet.

7. Enjoy while hot!

Alfredo The Chicken
Preparation 10 minutes || Cooking 30 minutes

Enjoy the flavor of succulent chicken breasts covered in a smooth, homemade Alfredo sauce. Mascarpone and Asiago cheeses give this version of our Carnivore Alfredo an additional layer of richness and flavor.

Ingredients :

- Two substantial organic chicken breasts
- 1/3 cup mascarpone cheese that is organic

- 3 tablespoons organic heavy cream for whipping
- 2 tablespoons grass-fed butter or Ghee
- -One teaspoon of salt
- Two tablespoons of organic Asiago shaved cheese

Add-Ins for Taste:

Add minced garlic, dried thyme, and freshly ground black pepper to the sauce for a more nuanced taste.

To Conserve Cash:

Choose bone-in chicken breasts and take out the meat from step 1's cooking.

Guidelines:

1. Place the chicken breasts in a large pot of boiling water. Cover and lower the heat to a minimum. Simmer until the chicken reaches an internal temperature of 165°F (74°C), about 20 minutes. Take off the heat and place aside.

2. Heat a medium-sized skillet and combine the butter, cream, mascarpone, and salt. After heating, turn down the heat to low and stir often for five minutes, or until the mixture thickens.

3. Using a fork, shred the chicken breasts, and use a knife to chop the skin. Mix the chicken thoroughly after adding the sauce.

4. While still hot, divide the chicken and sauce between two plates and top with Asiago cheese.

Turkey Breast In Brine
Preparation 10 minutes || Cooking 40- 50 minutes

Tear off the meat with your hands and teeth while holding a bone to savor the experience of eating like a primal. Just don't forget to carry napkins with you. You will need two cups of chicken broth, cooking fat, and bone-in chicken thighs for this recipe.

Cooking Advice: If a Dutch oven is not available, use a large, sturdy pot instead. Before putting it in the oven for step 6, make sure the pot is oven-proof.

Taste Add-ins: You can add some chopped onions and organic celery stalks to the dish to give the broth and meat some extra flavor.

Guidelines:

1. After adding salt, set the chicken thighs aside.

2. Prepare a Dutch oven.

3. The chicken thighs should be seared for 4 minutes, or until they are crisp and golden brown, with some butter heated in the pot. Flip them over and sear the other side after two minutes. After that, remove them and set them aside.

4. Deglaze the Dutch oven with the chicken broth.

5. Reintroduce the chicken into the saucepan. Add enough broth to cover halfway, turn down the heat, and cover.

6. Preheat the oven to 300°F (148°C). Cook the meat for an additional 30 minutes, or until a meat thermometer inserted into the thickest part, without touching the bone, reads 165°F (75°C). Alternatively, cook the meat until tender over low heat on the stove.

7. Allow the chicken to sit in its juices for a minimum of eight minutes before serving, then proceed to serve it warm.

Confit Of Duck
Preparation 15 minutes || Cooking 6-8 hours

Three essential elements of a successful meal are simplicity in preparation, intense flavor, and ease of cleanup. Duck is high in fat and protein and offers a nice variation to the diet.

Ingredients

Half a pound of duck fat, two whole breasts, and one tablespoon of salt

Flavor Enhancement: Drizzle cooked duck breasts with lemon juice and garnish with finely chopped parsley.

Guidelines:

1. Duck breasts should be put in a slow cooker. Add salt and fat.

2. After covering, cook for one hour on HIGH.

3. Simmer the duck for 4 to 8 hours, or until it is extremely tender, on LOW heat. To remove the duck from the fat, use a slotted spoon; the fat can be strained and used again.

4. Serve warm or hot duck.

Drumsticks With Salt
Preparation 10 minutes || Cooking 30 minutes

Lightly dust chicken drumsticks with coarse sea salt for a delightful crunch. The chicken will be crispy and hot. Serve them with your choice of Creamy Goat Cheese Sauce or Hollandaise as an appetizer or side dish.

Ingredients :

- 12 drumsticks of chicken raised without cages
- 1/2 cup of cooking fat (tallow, butter, ghee, or lard) that has melted
- Finely ground sea salt

Guidelines:

1. Set oven temperature to 450°F or 230°C.

2. Use parchment paper to line a baking sheet with a rim.

3. Combine the drumsticks and two tablespoons of cooking fat in a bowl.

4. Place the drumsticks on the baking sheet and bake until cooked through about 30 minutes. Halfway through cooking, brush them with the remaining 2 tablespoons of cooking fat.

5. Apply a generous amount of salt and broil for five minutes to achieve crispy skin. Maintain the food's warmth.

Crispy Thighs Of Chicken
Preparation 10 minutes || Cooking 35 minutes

You can eat the chicken thighs as soon as they're cool enough to handle. You will get oily palms from eating this delicious chicken thigh after just one bite.

Ingredients :

- Four organic, skin-on, bone-in chicken thighs
- 1/4 cup of cooking fat (lard, butter, ghee, or tallow) that has melted
- -Finely ground sea salt

Guidelines:

1. Set oven temperature to 450°F, or 230°C.

2. Place the chicken thighs in a cast-iron pan or skillet that is ovenproof. After basting with cooking fat, add salt for seasoning.

3. Bake the chicken thighs until they are cooked through, about 30 minutes.

4. Preheat the broiler and place the chicken under it for about five minutes to crisp the skin.

5. Always have plenty of napkins on hand, and serve hot.

Chicken Breast Wrapped In Prosciutto

Preparation 15 minutes || Cooking 25 minutes

A moist layer of thinly sliced prosciutto, or dry-cured Italian ham, envelops a cheese-filled chicken breast. The crispy baked texture of the aged meat offers a crunchy contrast to the juicy, soft chicken breast and oozy cheese.

Ingredients:

- 1 Tbsp. Heritage Pork Lard
- One-third cup of shredded organic Muenster cheese
- ½ cup of finely grated organic Parmesan cheese

- Two large free-range chicken breasts, butterflied and boneless
- Four thin yet thick pieces of fine prosciutto

Taste Add-ins: In step three, mix the cheese mixture with finely chopped fresh herbs like basil and thyme leaf.

Guidelines:

1. Turn the oven up to 400°F or 204°C.

2. Make sure the pan is evenly coated with heated lard in a large cast-iron or ovenproof skillet.

3. Take a bowl, mix the cheeses, cut them in half, and stuff each chicken breast evenly.

4. Encircle each chicken breast with two prosciutto slices.

5. After the prosciutto is crispy and the chicken reaches an internal temperature of at least 165°F (74°C), place the chicken breasts in the skillet and bake for about 25 minutes.

6. Season to taste, then add salt and serve hot.

Simmered Chicken Leg
Preparation 20 minutes || Cooking 45 minutes

Grab a bone and use your hands and teeth to pull off the meat to experience eating like a primal. Remember to always carry napkins!

Ingredients list:

- Four organic, free-range chicken thighs with the bone in
- A pair of cups of fat that has been cooked in chicken broth

Taste Add-ins: To enhance the flavor of the broth and meat, mix in some chopped onions and organic celery stalks.

Cooking Tip: In case you do not have a Dutch oven and want to move it to the oven in step 6, use a deep, heavy pot that is ovenproof.

Guidelines:

1. Before putting the chicken thighs aside, sprinkle them with salt.

2. Warm up a Dutch oven before adding butter. Once heated, sear the thighs for 4 minutes, skin-side down, or until they are crispy and browned. Flip it over after two minutes and sear the other side as well. Remove and set apart.

3. To deglaze the Dutch oven, use broth.

4. Reintroduce the chicken to the pot and cover it with broth halfway. Once you've brought it to a simmer, place a lid on it.

5. Continue cooking the meat in the preheated oven at 300°F (148°C) for an additional 30 minutes, or until a meat thermometer inserted into the thickest part, without touching the bone, registers 165°F (75°C). Alternatively, cook over low heat until the meat is very tender.

6. Serve warm, having soaked in the juices for at least eight minutes.

Chapter 5

EGG RECIPES

Peel-Able Boiling Eggs
Preparation 5 minutes || Cooking 15 minutes

Of all the methods for cooking eggs, this is my favorite for perfectly boiled eggs. Sea salt helps seal cracks and facilitates the peeling process. Depending on your preferences, you can make the eggs firm, medium-creamy, or soft and runny!

Ingredients:

- Eight free-range, organic eggs

Four or so cups of water

- One tsp unfiltered apple cider vinegar

- A single tablespoon of salt

Cooking Tips:

Based on "large" eggs that are regularly found in supermarkets, the timing was determined. Cooking times should be adjusted for smaller eggs.

Avoid Going Over Budget:

Before discarding old eggs, think about boiling them. A few days is the ideal age to boil eggs.

Guidelines:

1. Place the eggs in a pan with a single layer on the bottom and add enough water to cover by at least one inch.

2. Add the salt and vinegar to the water and stir gently.

3. Once you've brought the water to a boil, use the timer to gauge the desired doneness (see the times listed on the page facing you). Don't cover it with a lid.

4. After the specified amount of time has passed, remove the pot from the hot water and immerse it in cold running water. Let it run until the water gets very cold, which may take a few minutes.

5. Let the eggs sit at room temperature for ten minutes.

6. Until the eggs' shell is covered in cracks, gently roll them around and tap them on a

countertop. Once removed, the shell should come off easily under running water!

7. Eggs that have been peeled should be consumed immediately, and eggs that are still in their shell can be kept in the refrigerator for about a week. Steer clear of freezing.

Fried Eggs With Butter Basting
Preparation 1 minute || Cooking 5 minutes

Baste the eggs with warm fat to ensure that the whites cook quickly without sacrificing the yolks' moisture content. The high heat causes the egg whites to crisp up while the yolks stay gooey and soft. This is the best fried egg recipe, in our opinion.

Ingredients :

- Three tsp of butter from grass-fed cattle
- Four free-range, organic eggs
- Salt

Guidelines:

1. Melt the butter in a skillet over medium-high heat until it shimmers.

2. One egg at a time, carefully add it to the pan, being careful not to splash yourself. Add a little salt to taste.

3. To get the butter to gather on the side, tilt the skillet in your direction. Using a spoon, drizzle warm butter over the eggs, being careful to coat the whites only, not the yolk.

4. Baste the eggs for 45–60 seconds, or until they are puffed and cooked. Place on a platter and serve warm.

Easy Farmhouse Eggs
Preparation 1 minute || Cooking 5 minutes

On days when you want a hot breakfast but don't want to spend a lot of time cooking and cleaning, this recipe is ideal.

Ingredients :
- Four free-range, organic eggs
- Two teaspoons of fat for cooking
- Salt

Cooking Tip: Depending on how many eggs you have, cut the egg whites in half with a spatula to make flipping easier.

Guidelines:

1. Melt the fat in a skillet over medium heat, and crack the eggs into a side bowl.

2. Add the eggs to the pan once the fat begins to sizzle. To enable the eggs to gather on the far side of the skillet, tilt the skillet by lifting the handle. Allow to cook for 30 seconds, or until the edge of the whites starts to form a crust.

3. Lower the handle and lay the pan flat. Cook for a further fifteen seconds, moving the pan slightly to keep it from sticking. To taste, add salt. Cook for one minute on low heat.

4. Turn the eggs with a spatula once the whites are set but not firm. Cook for an additional fifteen seconds, then turn them over to the other side. After moving to a platter, serve warm.

Eggs Scrambled In A Diner Style
Preparation 1 minute || Cooking 5 minutes

Overcooking scrambled eggs can cause them to become dry, rubbery, or resemble omelets. Enjoy your nutritious, quick, and simple dinner of scrambled eggs as soon as possible.

Ingredients :

- Three free-range, organic eggs
- A teaspoon of cooking oil or unsalted butter
- Optional one tablespoon of organic sour cream
- One-half teaspoon salt

Add-ons For Taste: Add iodine-rich seaweeds, like dulse or wakame flakes, on top for more flavor and minerals.

Guidelines:

1. Pour the butter and cracked eggs into a cold, ungreased pan.

2. Heat the stove to medium-high and whisk the eggs and butter together with a spatula.

3. Until the eggs are cooked through, keep stirring.

4. Season with salt and optional sour cream. Place on a platter and serve warm.

Lorraine's Crusted Quiche
Preparation 10 minutes || Cooking 30 minutes

Eggs, smoky Gruyère cheese, and flavorful bacon combine to create the incredibly light and creamy dish known as crustless quiche Lorraine. Serve it to guests; it's a delightful and satisfying brunch or breakfast option!

Ingredients :
- A single pound of raw bacon
- Four free-range, organic eggs
- 1/4 cup heavy cream, organic
- ½ cup of shredded organic Gruyère cheese

- A teaspoon of salt

Add-ins for taste:

Step 4: Add some chopped onion, dill, and smoked salmon to the egg mixture.

Guidelines:

1. Preheat the oven to 350°F/175°C and lightly grease a pie pan.

2. In a large skillet, cook the bacon for approximately six minutes. Store the grease in a jar and leave it on a side plate to cool. Chop the bacon into small pieces.

3. In a large bowl, beat together the eggs and cream.

4. Mix the cheese, bacon, and salt thoroughly into the eggs.

5. Spoon the mixture into a lightly oiled pie dish and bake for 20 minutes, or until the center is set.

6. Before slicing and serving, give it a five-minute rest.

Eggs Baked Softly
Preparation 5 minutes || Cooking 15 minutes

This easy recipe keeps well in the fridge, is great for the whole family, and makes a great batch meal. Put these egg cups in your children's lunchboxes or serve them to them after school.

Ingredients :

- Applying cooking fat to a muffin pan
- Twelve large eggs, free-range and organic.
- A teaspoon of salt

Cooking tips:

For a perfectly gooey yolk, cook until the cooking time reaches about 12 minutes.

Refrain from making purchases:
These are far superior to any store-bought snack for hungry kids. Put them in the fridge to take the place of chips and crackers.

Guidelines:
1. Preheat the oven to 175°C (350°F).
2. Grease a standard-size 12-cup muffin pan.
3. Make sure not to break the yolks by carefully cracking an egg into each muffin cup.
4. Season with salt, if desired.

5. The egg whites should be baked for 12 to 15 minutes, or until set. Remove from the oven and allow to sit for a few minutes, then loosen the sides with a knife. Leftovers can be consumed warm or cold.

Eggs Scotch
Preparation 15 minutes || Cooking 25 minutes

Supermarkets, corner stores, and gas stations carry Scotch eggs, a favorite picnic food. They are usually found in the UK and consist of a layer of sausage wrapped around boiled eggs.

Ingredients :

- Two pounds of ground pork that is organic
- two teaspoons of salt
- 12 large, peeled, boiled organic free-range eggs

Ready in bulk:

You could easily double or triple the recipe if you'd like. It stores well and fits neatly into everyone's lunchbox.

Guidelines:

1. Preheat the oven to 175°C (350°F).

2. Line two rimmed baking sheets with parchment paper.

3. Combine the pork and the salt in a large bowl. Using your hands, combine the ingredients to form 12 meatballs. Place and press six meatballs flat on each of the baking sheets that have been lined.

4. Place one hard-boiled egg in the center of each meat round, making sure that it is completely surrounded by no gaps or openings.

5. Bake for about 15 minutes. After that, turn them over and continue baking for ten more minutes, or until the outside is nicely browned. Finish under the broiler for five minutes for a crispy shell. Reheat the meal.

Omelet Stuffed With Swordfish
Preparation 5 minutes || Cooking 5 minutes

Any type of homemade protein can be layered into eggs along with cheese for seasoning. Try leftovers like simple baked salmon, slow-cooked beef brisket, or chicken Alfredo in place of swordfish.

Ingredients :

- Three free-range, organic eggs
- 1 tablespoon cooking oil or unsalted butter
- One cup of leftover oven-roasted swordfish with a salt and smoke crust
- Optional: Shredded organic cheese

Guidelines:

1. Beat the eggs in a small bowl.

2. Cooking fat should be heated to a medium temperature in a skillet.

3. Pour the eggs into the hot pan. As they harden, raise the edges to allow the raw material to flow underneath.

4. Once cooked, remove from the heat but do not remove the eggs from the pan. Place the fish on top of a half of an egg. Add the cheese, if desired. Fold the omelet over to conceal the filling.

5. Serve immediately, or cover the pan and let it sit for a minute to melt the cheese if using it. Place on a platter and serve warm.

Egg And Bacon Scramble Cups
Preparation 15 minutes || Cooking 35 minutes

Here, two staple breakfast ingredients—bacon and eggs—combine to create a filling, finger-food recipe. These cups have cheese on top and are "crusted" with bacon. Serve as single servings or put in lunchboxes for the entire workweek.

Ingredients:

- 18 slices of uncured bacon
- Ten organic free-range eggs
- One cup of heavy whipping cream, organic
- One tsp salt
- ½ cup cheese, shredded organically

Guidelines:

1. Set the oven's temperature to 175°C/350°F. 2. Line each muffin cup with a slice of bacon, enclosing it around the edges.

3. Chop the remaining six bacon strips into 2-inch segments. To create a floor, place two pieces in the bottom of each cup. Entirety cover the bottom.

4. In a bowl, whisk together the eggs, cream, and salt. 5. Evenly pour the egg mixture into every well. Tops with cheese sprinkled over them.

6. Bake until golden brown, about 35 minutes. Take off the heat, let it cool, then serve it warm. Keep any leftovers chilled.

Breakfast Cereal

Breakfast Cereal
Preparation 15 minutes || Cooking 30 minutes

You can create a satisfying, low-carb, gluten-free casserole that's ideal for a meat lover with ground meat, eggs, cream, and cheese. This recipe can be doubled and kept in a 9x13 dish for several days, so it's also a great option for dinner or breakfast.

Ingredients :

- One pound of ground beef, sausage, or leftover slow-cooked meat from bison
- Six large eggs, free-range and organic.

- 1/2 cup organic heavy whipping cream
- A pair of teaspoons of homemade cream cheese
- A teaspoon of salt

Guidelines:

1. Warm up the oven to 190°C, or 375°F.

2. Gently brown the meat in a skillet over medium heat for about 5 minutes, stirring often to break up any clumps.

3. Lightly beat the eggs in a medium-sized bowl, then stir in the cream cheese, salt, and cream. Next, incorporate the meat thoroughly.

4. Fill a 9-inch shallow pie dish with the egg-meat mixture and brush with cooking fat. Bake for 20 to 25 minutes, until the

eggs are set and the pie's top is browned. After letting it rest for ten minutes, slice it and serve.

Carnivorous Salad
Preparation 5 minutes || Cooking 5 minutes

This dinner is entirely my spouse's fault because he combined two of his favorite foods, canned sardines, and fried eggs, into a single bowl. To observe the subtle differences in effects between flavors, experiment with different types of salt.

Ingredients :

- Three butter-battered fried eggs
- A single 4.75-ounce can of wild sardines in a solution
- A teaspoon of salt

Guidelines:

1. Once the eggs are ready, transfer them to a bowl and, after the can is opened, add the heated sardines to the eggs.

2. Stir well after adding the salt. To taste, add extra butter. Serve immediately.

3. Give a hug to Tristan.

Love Cheese Bacon Frittatas
Preparation 10 minutes || Cooking 30 minutes

Bacon and eggs are elevated to a whole new level in this cheesy frittata that includes bacon, meat, eggs, cream, and cheese. It's a tasty, creamy, low-fiber dish.

Ingredients:

- Eight ounces of uncured, center-cut bacon
- Eight ounces of organic ground pork
- Eight large eggs, free-range and organic
- 1/2 cup organic heavy whipping cream
- 1/2 cup organically shredded cheese
- A teaspoon of salt

- Your favorite low-carb veggies and a dash of black pepper (optional)

Guidelines:

1. Set oven temperature to 175°C/350°F.

2. Elevate the temperature in an ovenproof skillet to medium-high. When the bacon is crispy, cook it for three to four minutes on each side. Remove and allow to cool.

3. Brown the pork using the leftover bacon fat. Break up any clumps with a wooden spatula and cook for about 5 minutes. Remove the meat with a slotted spoon and set it aside to cool.

4. Beat the eggs in a medium-sized mixing bowl. To the eggs, add the crumbled pork and bacon. Stir in the cream, cheese, and salt.

5. Pour the whisked eggs into the skillet and bake until the top is browned and the eggs are set about 20 minutes. Before slicing, turn off the stove and give it ten minutes to rest.

Traditional Pickled Eggs
Preparation 5 minutes || Cooking 5 minutes

English taverns have served pickled eggs as a popular dish since the 1830s. This nutrient-dense bar snack, popularized by German saloons in America, is usually found submerged in vinegar jars on the counter.

Ingredients :

- A teaspoon of salt
- Eight boiled eggs that are easy to peel.
- One cup of water and half a cup of raw apple cider vinegar

- One teaspoon of pickling spices, dried herbs, or cloves of garlic (optional)

Guidelines:

1. Put salt in a glass jar that holds one liter.

2. Pour in the vinegar and water, and stir to combine.

3. Place the peeled eggs inside the jar.

4. After covering it, leave it in the fridge for two days.

5. If desired, add a dash of salt as a garnish.

Breakfast Muffins With No Fiber
Preparation 10 minutes || Cooking 20 minutes

When baking breakfast muffins, eggs and different ground meats (beef, beef heart, pork, chicken, bison, or lamb) work great.

Ingredients :

- Cooking fat
- Nine large eggs, free-range and organic.
- A single teaspoon of salt
- Eight ounces of grass-fed ground beef

Flavoring Add-ins:

Step 4's eggs are simple to incorporate with sautéed onions, garlic, mushrooms, and herbs.

Guidelines:

1. Adjust the oven's heat setting to 350°F/175°C.

2. Grease a standard-size muffin pan with your preferred cooking fat.

3. In a skillet over medium heat, brown the meat.

4. Add the meat and salt to a large bowl with the whisked eggs and stir to combine.

5. Before you pour the batter into the muffin tins, fill ¾ of each muffin cup with batter. Bake the eggs for 20 minutes to set them.

6. Remove the muffins from the oven, allow them to cool for five minutes, let them open with a knife, and serve warm or store them in the fridge for later use.

Benedict Eggs And Beef
Preparation 5 minutes || Cooking 5minutes

Make a fiery carnivore eggs Benedict with slow-cooked goat leg in broth or slow-cooked meat from bone broth:

Ingredients :
- Two free-range, organic eggs
- One teaspoon vinegar
- 1/4 cup of beef cooked slowly
- One serving of Hollandaise sauce

Cooking Tip:
You have the option of poaching the whole egg or just the yolk. Save the whites for

making frothy milk by whisking them with warm milk.

Guidelines:

1. Pour vinegar into a small pot of simmering water.

2. Crack eggs into a bowl, taking care not to crack the yolks.

3. Simmer the water gently with the eggs in it, poaching them for three minutes.

4. When the meat is cooked through in a skillet, move it to a platter.

5. The poached eggs can be removed and placed over the meat bed using a slotted spoon.

6. Drizzle the eggs with the Hollandaise Sauce, serve immediately, and enjoy warm.

No-churn Ingredients

Preparation 10 minutes || Cooking 4 Hours

Cream and egg yolks should be carefully whisked together to create a delicious homemade ice cream. Visit farmers' markets to sample local honey that varies slightly in flavor according to the season.

Ingredients:

- Egg yolks, four to six
- A single liter of raw dairy cream
- Unprocessed honey from the area

Cooking Tip: Use an immersion blender with a whisk attachment to combine the egg and cream mixture in a freezer-safe container (such as a mason jar) to minimize cleanup. After that, immediately put the mixture in cold storage.

Add-ins For Flavor: To improve the flavor, start with a ¼ teaspoon of extract and taste as you go. Some examples of extracts to try are vanilla, mint, or lemon. You can also use liquid monkfruit sweetener if you'd like.

Guidelines:

1. Beat the cream and the egg yolks together.

2. With a hand mixer or an electric whisk, mix for thirty to sixty seconds.

3. Place the mixture in a freezer-safe container, cover, and freeze for at least four hours.

4. Remove from the freezer ten to fifteen minutes before serving.

5. Serve by scooping and then dousing with a spoonful or two of honey.

Chapter 6

SOURCES & FATS

Ghee
Preparation 20 minutes || Cooking 15 minutes

Make ghee first, then use it to make a versatile homemade cooking oil that tastes great with meat, fish, and eggs. Ghee, which is made by clarifying butter to remove milk solids, is often tolerated by those who are intolerant to dairy products. In Ayurvedic traditions, ghee is highly valued for its digestive qualities.

Ingredients: - 1 cup unsalted grass-fed butter

Cooking Tip: Consider flavoring your food with the leftover milk solids from the clarification process for your upcoming meal.

Historical Note: Ghee, an integral part of Indian culture, has long been made from the milk of water buffaloes. Due to its ceremonial and health-promoting properties, it was widely traded and held great value. Folktales, religious rites, and national hymns all extolled it.

Guidelines:

1. Chop the butter into small pieces and add it to a small saucepan over low heat.

2. Once the butter has melted, increase the heat so that it cooks. When the water boils off, a layer of white foam will form on the surface.

3. Cook for about ten minutes, watching closely to make sure the bottom of the pan with the milk solids is browning.

4. Switch off the heat source and give it a ten-minute rest.

5. Carefully strain the liquid into a clean glass jar using a fine-mesh sieve covered in two layers of cheesecloth.

6. Once cooled, cover and store in the refrigerator for up to six months, or freeze for longer storage.

Tallow In The Pioneer Style
Preparation 30 minutes || Cooking 4-6 Hours

The solid white fat called suet covers the kidneys and loins of animals such as sheep and cattle. For superior quality, it is advised to choose suet from ruminants that have been fed grass. This fat keeps well in storage for extended periods and is ideal for high-temperature cooking. This is how to prepare tallow in your own home:

Ingredients :

- Four lbs of sweet suet

Guidelines:

1. Finely chop the white, waxy fat and place it over very low heat in an empty stockpot.

2. Place a lid on the pot and create a tiny opening to let heat or steam out. Cook, stirring occasionally to avoid burning, for 4–6 hours.

3. When impurities and oil bubbles rise to the top, tallow is created.

4. After a brief cooling period, strain the mixture through a fine mesh strainer lined with cheesecloth. Keep the bits of suet for cracklings.

5. For extended storage, place in the refrigerator or store in a glass jar at room temperature for a few months.

Vintage Pork Fat
Preparation 20 minutes || Cooking 2 Hours

Pie crusts frequently contain lard, a hidden ingredient that improves baked goods' texture. If overdone, though, it could make desserts taste too "piggy." This is how to prepare lard in your own home:

Ingredients:

- 1/2 cup water to

- 2 ½ pounds heritage hog fat or leaf lard-bred hog

Guidelines:

1. Cut the pork fat into small pieces to remove any large pieces of meat or blood.

2. Transfer chopped pork fat to a crockpot, pour ½ cup water over it, and reduce the heat to low. Simmer, stirring occasionally, until the fat melts and the cracklings rise to the top, about 2 hours.

3. Allow to cool slightly before straining the fat through a cheesecloth-lined colander into a glass jar or jars. Store in the refrigerator, freezer, or at a cool room temperature if not using right away.

Oleic acid and vitamin D are two important nutrients found in lard.

Duck Fat

Preparation 1 Hour || Cooking 15 minutes

In Southwest France, duck fat is a staple ingredient that gives food flavor and texture. This is how to prepare duck fat in your kitchen:

Ingredients :

- Fat from geese or ducks
- Water

Guidelines:

1. Transfer the duck fat to a frying pan after coarsely chopping it.

2. Add water to the pan and cook over medium heat, stirring, until the fat is dissolved.

3. Continue cooking until there is just a light simmer and no more water visible.

4. Filter out the duck fat, reserving the pieces for cracklings.

5. Transfer the duck fat to a glass jar, let it come to room temperature, and keep it in the freezer for up to a year or the refrigerator for up to six months.

Crackers
Preparation 5 minutes || Cooking 5 minutes

Make delicious garnishes out of leftover suet or animal fat with crispy cracklings. How to make them at home is as follows:

Ingredients:

- Scraps of suet, duck fat, or lard left over from tallow making
- Salt

Add-ons: To give your popcorn a unique flavor, mix in some nutritional yeast or herb salt. Serve it separately or drizzle it over the salad.

Guidelines:

1. Strain duck fat, lard, or tallow; collect any leftover fat fragments.

2. In a skillet over low heat, fry for about five minutes, or until crispy, browned, and completely dry. Avoid lighting them on fire!

3. Sprinkle a generous amount of salt on top of the hot dish.

Veloute with Brown Butter

It takes five minutes to prepare and twenty minutes to cook this recipe.

Veloute

A broth base is used to make veloute, a sauce that can be made with fish, poultry, or veal. With its deep flavor and abundance of good fats, this sauce is a fantastic complement to any meat dish. To meals like pan-seared pork chops, steamed mussels, and slow-cooked meat, browned butter adds a deep, rich flavor.

Ingredients :
- 1/4 cup butter made from grass
- 1/4 cup organic heavy cream for whipping

- ¼ cup chicken broth from free-range chicken - 1 teaspoon salt

Guidelines:

1. Brown the butter in a pan over medium heat for up to ten minutes, swirling occasionally.

2. Combine the browned butter, cream, broth, and salt in a small saucepan.

3. Stir everything thoroughly and lower the heat to a simmer.

4. Continue stirring until the sauce thickens, which should take another five to ten minutes. Before serving, reheat the food.

Blended Butters
Preparation 1 minutes || Cooking 0 minutes

To add even more flavor, experiment with different herbs and spices. Use parsley, thyme, oregano, or a combination of them. Mix these flavors with salt and softened butter to make a versatile compound butter.

Ingredients:

- ½ cup of softened butter from grass-fed cows
- The organic herbs and spices of your choice
- One teaspoon of salt

Add-ins For Flavor:

- 1 tablespoon minced basil and ½ head roasted garlic - 2 ounces blue cheese and 1 minced clove garlic

- 4 ounces of goat cheese that has softened and minced chives

Guidelines:

1. Combine salt, butter, and a few chosen flavors in a medium-sized mixing bowl.

2. Place plastic wrap over the surface of your work.

3. Roll up the plastic wrap and twist the outer edges to seal the butter into a 6-inch log.

4. Before serving, let the butter cool in the refrigerator for at least two hours. Use cold

slices as a garnish on hot dishes or as a stuffing for broiled burgers.

Fat Taste Infusion
Preparation 5 minutes || Cooking 4-6 hours

Beef tallow, pork lard, duck fat, and butter are all great vehicles for incorporating herbs and spices. To prevent spoiling, use dried herbs or spice blends rather than fresh ones. Some delectable options include infused boneless pork chops seared in lard, infused butter-basted fried eggs, and infused beef burgers cooked in tallow.

Ingredients:

- Any organic spices and herbs of your choice

- Half a cup of melted cooking oil

Addition Of Flavor: nutmeg, ginger powder, and ground cinnamon
- Ground black pepper and turmeric powder - Mint and lemon zest
- Powdered vanilla and cinnamon

Cooking Tip: To achieve a smoother infusion, strain the fat from the herbs after the infusion period. Throw away the herbs.

Guidelines:
1. Transfer fat to the top of a clean glass jar filled with herbs.

2. Simmer the jar over low heat for four to six hours in a small saucepan filled with water.

3. Check the water levels regularly and add more room-temperature water as needed.

4. Allow the jar to cool before using it immediately, or store it in the refrigerator or another cold, dark place. The date and ingredient labels should be attached. Store out of direct sunlight. Use within a month for optimal outcomes.

Cheddar Fries
Preparation 5 minutes || Cooking 5 minutes

Provolone, queso blanco, paneer, and halloumi can all be fried to golden perfection. Alternately, pile cheese shreds into small mounds in a pan and flip them over as soon as they start to bubble. Cook, stirring, until crispy, making a tasty snack.

Ingredients:
- 4 tablespoons cooking fat
- 4 ounces cheese, any kind - Salt

Guidelines:
1. Cut the cheese into ½-inch cubes.

2. Reheat cooking fat in a frying pan over medium–high heat.

3. Carefully add the cheese to the pan when the oil starts to spew. There will be bubbles in the cheese.

4. Cook, rotating once or twice to ensure even cooking, for three to five minutes. Once the cheese is plated, sprinkle it with salt and serve it hot or warm.

Alfredo Carnivore
Preparation 5 minutes || Cooking 10 minutes

Make a carnivorous Alfredo sauce with just what's required to maintain the beloved classic flavor. For a flavorful twist, drizzle over prosciutto-wrapped chicken breast or sautéed sliced steak.

Ingredients:
- One tablespoon of grass-fed cow's butter
- 1/2 cup of grated Parmesan cheese
- 1/2 cup of organic heavy cream for whipping
- Salt

Cooking Tip: If you prefer a thinner sauce, gradually add extra cream after step 3 to get the desired texture.

Guidelines:

1. In a small saucepan over medium heat, melt the butter.

2. Reduce the volume by one-third after adding the cream. Simmer for about five minutes on low heat, or until sauce thickens.

3. Reduce the temperature. Whisk in the Parmesan cheese gradually until smooth. Season and add salt to taste. Reheat the meal.

Goat Cheese Spread
Preparation 10 minutes || Cooking 10 minutes

This adaptable sauce complements a wide range of seafood and meats. Use it as a dressing for a delicious carnivorous dish, or to coat Crispy Chicken Thighs and dip Scotch Eggs.

Ingredients:
- 2 tsp butter from grass-fed cow
- 1/4 cup heavy whipping cream that is organic
- 1/4 cup soft goat cheese; - 1/4 cup grated aged goat cheese
- Salt

Cooking Tip: You can use more cream or water to thin the sauce. Alternatively, to achieve a thicker consistency, cook it for an additional three to five minutes.

Guidelines:

1. In a small saucepan, preheat the cream and butter.

2. Include the soft cheese, stir well, and cook over low heat until bubbling.

3. As soon as bubbles start to form, turn off the heat. Add grated cheese and stir until smooth and creamy. After adding salt, serve.

Homemade Sour Cream
Preparation 5 minutes || Cooking 4-6 Hours

Use raw cream to naturally sour it overnight, or infuse pasteurized cream with exogenous bacteria to create a probiotic-rich product. When using pasteurized cream, stay away from using ultra-high temperature processed (UHT) cream.

Ingredients:

To inoculate, use store-bought sour cream:

- Three cups organic heavy whipping cream, either raw or pasteurized.

- One cup of store-bought live cultured sour cream

To inoculate, use a starting culture:
- Four cups of raw or pasteurized heavy cream
- 1/8 teaspoon of direct-set sour cream culture or 1 packet of mesophilic starter culture

Shopping Tip: For a variety of starter cultures and supplies, visit the Cultures for Health website.

Guidelines:

1. Heat the cream to 86°F (30°C) and stir in the sour cream or starter culture.

2. To allow some air to circulate while keeping bugs out, transfer to a bowl or mason jar and cover loosely with a towel or cheesecloth.

3. Allow the cream to sit at room temperature for a period of 12 to 24 hours, or until it becomes thicker and flavorful with tang.

4. Serve immediately or, for additional slow fermentation, store in the refrigerator in an airtight container.

Homemade Cream Cheese
Preparation 5 minutes || Cooking 12 Hours

This recipe for cream cheese is ideal for spreading over slices of roast beef or liver crisps. Opt for pasteurized or raw cream instead of UHT-processed cream. Customize the flavor by adding fresh berries, herbs, or spices in the final step.

Ingredients:

1/8 teaspoon mesophilic starter culture;
4 cups raw or pasteurized organic heavy whipping cream

Shopping Tip: Visit your neighborhood health food stores or place an online order for a mesophilic culture from Cultures for Health.

Flavor Add-ins: In the final stages, add spices, herbs, or fresh berries to improve the flavor.

Guidelines:

1. In a glass bowl, gently stir the starter culture into the cream.

2. Let it stand, covered loosely with a towel or cheesecloth, at room temperature for a minimum of 12 to 18 hours, or until it takes on the consistency of yogurt.

3. Pour the thickened cream into a bowl and cover it with a cheesecloth-lined colander. Give the whey at least 12 hours to

drip out. The longer the whey separates, the harder the cheese becomes.

4. Once the cheese reaches the proper consistency, transfer it to an airtight container. If you want to season, add salt. As it cools, the cheese will continue to solidify.

3-Step Gravy Sauce Without Flour
Preparation 5 minutes || Cooking 5 minutes

For best results, serve the gravy hot and enjoy it right away. Simply reheat and whisk until smooth if it becomes thick as it cools. Depending on your tastes, you can also add bulk sausage or cooked ground beef to the gravy. Use butter in place of the lard to make a version without pork. Serve Braised Chuck Roast or Brined Turkey Breast with this aromatic gravy.

Ingredients :

- Two tablespoons of natural halves

- One tablespoon of warm water
Homemade Cream Cheese in the Country
- One tablespoon of Heritage Pork Fat
A couple of tablespoons of water
- Salt

Cooking Tip: Instead of using water to thin the gravy, use broth if any is available.

Guidelines:

1. Heat the half-and-half with the cream cheese and lard in a small saucepan over medium heat, whisking until smooth.

2. Gradually add water until the right consistency is achieved.

3. Season with salt to taste. Perfect with some meat.

Hollandaise Sauce
Preparation 5 minutes || Cooking 10 minutes

The classic sauce's creamy, buttery goodness. Feel free to replace the apple cider vinegar with lemon juice for a tangier twist. Serve with Beef and Eggs Benedict, Broiled Salmon Fillets, or Bacon-Wrapped Sea Bass.

Ingredients:
 - Half a cup of grass-fed butter
 - Three free-range egg yolks
One-fourth cup unrefined apple cider vinegar; one-half teaspoon optional cayenne or paprika

Cooking Tip: For a traditional hollandaise sauce with a kick, add cayenne pepper. For a simpler, tangier sauce, omit it.

Chapter 7

SEAFOOD AND FISH

Carnivorous Crab Dip
Preparation 5 minutes || Cooking 30 minutes

Savor this dip by itself or with optional vegetable sticks or crackers. Eat it with crispy bacon strips, liver crisps, or ground heart crunchies.

Ingredients:

- One teaspoon of salt

- One cup of country home cream cheese at room temperature
- One pound of meat lump crab

Flavor Add-ins: Experiment with different kinds of salt, like smoky sea salt or black lava salt.

Notable Nutrients: This amazingly creamy dip is packed with copper, vitamin B12, selenium, omega-3 fatty acids, and other trace minerals.

Guidelines:

1. Set oven temperature to 450°F, or 230°C.
2. Apply butter grease to a small baking dish.

3. Mix the cream cheese, salt, and crab meat together in a mixing bowl.

4. Once in the baking dish, transfer the mixture and bake for thirty minutes. Reheat and proceed to serve.

Steaming Mussels
Preparation 10 minutes || Cooking 30 minutes

Mussels are a delectable alternative to seafood that tastes especially good in the winter. Purchase them fresh, and consider collecting them yourself from the sea if you are able.

Ingredients :

- Two pounds of freshly cleaned, scrubbed, and debearded mussels
- Salt (optional)
Grass-based butter (optional)

Guidelines:

1. Place the mussels in a large bowl and cover with cold water.

2. In a pot large enough to hold the mussels, bring the water to a boil.

3. Once the water is boiling, place the mussels in it, cover it, and cook for 8 to 10 minutes, shaking the pot occasionally to make sure the mussels are thoroughly cooked.

4. Pour the mussels into a colander to cool, discarding any that haven't opened. Serve hot and garnish with butter and salt, if desired.

Simple Seared Salmon
Preparation 5 minutes || Cooking 10 minutes

Include some succulent, nutrient-dense wild-caught salmon in your weekly meal preparation schedule. Select local, fresh sources when they are available.

Ingredients :

- Split a half-cup of Ghee

- One teaspoon of salt

- Four 6-oz wild salmon filets

Cooking Tip: To make this recipe dairy-free, you can also use duck fat or flavor-infused fat.

Guidelines:

1. Set oven temperature to 450°F, or 230°C.

2. In a cast-iron skillet or oven-safe skillet, melt two tablespoons of butter over medium heat. Add salt and stir.

3. Once the oil is heated, place the salmon fillets skin-side down. Once one minute has passed, flip and sear the other side for a further minute.

4. After moving the skillet inside the oven, top it with the remaining 2 tablespoons. For eight minutes, bake. Servings hot are advised.

Cod Baked in Butter
Preparation 5 minutes || Cooking 20
minutes

Cod has long been a mainstay in many cultures' diets. This particular kind of fish flakes easily, has a mild flavor, and is an ocean-dwelling species. For more than a millennium, dried cod has been a prized commodity in Southern European trade, and its continued presence poses a serious risk to the Norwegian fishing sector.

Ingredients :
- Four 6-oz filets of cod
- Sea salt
- 1/4 cup pasture butter or ghee

Notable Nutrients: Rich in bioavailable vitamins A, D, and E as well as the fatty acids EPA and DHA, fermented cod liver oil and cod livers are highly prized. Both are regarded as important foods from the past.

Cooking Tip: Haddock or pollock can be substituted for cod if you don't have any.

Guidelines:

1. Set oven temperature to 400°F, or 204°C.
2. Salt the fish fillets on both sides for seasoning.
3. Transfer the fillets to a baking dish and coat each one with a tablespoon of butter or ghee.

4. The fish should flake easily with a fork after 20 minutes in the oven.

5. Gather any pan drippings after the fillets are plated and spoon them over the fillets. Warm up the food.

Seared Filets Of Salmon
Preparation 10 minutes || Cooking 10 minutes

Some fishing companies deliver Alaskan wild-caught salmon at a discount during certain seasons. You can look into your options for directly sourcing or signing up for subscription services.

Ingredients :

- Four filets of wild salmon
- 1/4 cup of ghee, melted
- Salt

Cooking Tip: To make this recipe dairy-free, replace the butter or ghee with duck fat or any other preferred cooking fat.

Guidelines:

1. After transferring the salmon filets to a level glass or enamel dish, completely coat them with melted ghee by brushing over them.

2. Activate the broiler.

3. Place the filets 3 inches below the heat source and broil for about 6 minutes. Gently turn them over, and if necessary, brush with additional butter. For an extra four minutes, broil. Season with salt and serve warm.

Tacos With Shrimp
Preparation 5 minutes || Cooking 10 minutes

These soft and crunchy shrimp tacos would be great for breakfast, lunch, or dinner. These make a great first course or snack when shared around the kitchen island.

Ingredients :

- Half a cup of Colby cheese, shredded
- Half a cup of cheddar cheese, shredded
- 1/2 cup of Monterey Jack cheese, shredded
- For the shrimp, use 1/2 tablespoon of grass-fed butter or ghee.

– Ten medium-sized shrimp, deveined and peeled

Cooking Tip: If you'd rather make another seafood dish, you can replace the shrimp with leftover boiled salmon or butter-baked cod.

Guidelines:

1. Adjust the oven temperature to 350°F (175°C) and place parchment paper on a baking sheet.

2. In a bowl, combine the three cheeses; shape into six rounds, each measuring four inches, to place on the baking sheet. Bake until browned, about 5 minutes.

3. Before using a spatula to form the cheese rounds into taco shells, let them

cool slightly. While they cool, turn them over and reshape them as necessary.

4. Shrimp should be cooked for 5 to 7 minutes, or until they turn pink, in butter or ghee over medium heat. Before slicing them into smaller pieces, let them cool.

5. Serve the warm shrimp by dividing them equally among the taco shells.

Steaming Fish
Preparation 10 minutes || Cooking 25 minutes

Although carp is widely used in Asian cooking, it is also common in fresh, eutrophic lakes and big rivers in the USA and Europe. Serve this warm fish with a slice of compound butter or a bowl of brown butter Veloute and squeeze some lemon juice over it.

Ingredients :

- A single, four to five-pound carp
- Warm water

Cooking Tip: Use a steamer basket inside a large pot with water in the bottom for smaller portions of fish. You should adjust the cooking time for one-pound filets, as they can steam for less than ten minutes.

Guidelines:

1. Before putting the fish on a rack over hot water, scale and clean it using a turkey roaster or a homemade arrangement.

2. When the water reaches a rolling boil, reduce the heat and simmer the fish, covered tightly, for 25 minutes, or until it flakes easily with a fork.

3. Serve hot or warm.

Seared Abalone Filets
Preparation 5 minutes || Cooking 10 minutes

Living on the Northern California coast, my aunt frequently goes abalone diving in the Pacific. When we get together as a family, we discuss the catch of the day, and abalone is always the most popular dish. This is how to cook abalone:

Ingredients :

- Two sizable, ¼-inch-thick abalone steaks

- A quarter cup of melted ghee (or your favorite cooking fat)

- Salt

To enhance the taste, consider adding sautéed garlic, lime juice, minced cilantro, or homemade sour cream.

Guidelines:

1. Tenderize the steaks to a ¼-inch thickness with a wooden mallet.

2. Heat ghee or cooking fat in a skillet over medium heat.

3. The abalone steaks should be cooked in the melted fat for 30 seconds on each side.

4. Season with salt and serve right away.

Easy Baked Salmon
Preparation 10 minutes || Cooking 25 minutes

Fish baking is an essential culinary skill. This versatile recipe works well for baking any type of fish. Using a spoon or basting tool, remove any extra fat or butter from the top by sprinkling it on several times while baking.

The recipe is as follows:

Ingredients :

- Half a cup of ghee, or your preferred cooking fat

- Two pounds of wild salmon, either fillets or steaks

Add some finely sliced white onion rings, some fresh dill sprigs, and a squeeze of lemon juice as flavoring additions.

Guidelines:

1. Preheat the oven to 400°F, or 204°C.

2. In a small skillet, melt the ghee or cooking fat until it starts to turn golden. To guarantee an even coating, swirl the browned fat into a 9 x 13-inch baking dish. Include the salmon in the recipe.

3. Bake, baste frequently, for twenty-five minutes on the salmon. The fish is done when a fork flakes through it with ease. Bake times should be adjusted for thicker pieces.

4. After seasoning, add salt to taste and serve hot.

Smoked Trout
Preparation 5 minutes || Cooking 10 minutes

A great option for a weeknight or last-minute dinner is trout, which is infused with a delightful smokiness and gets warm and crispy under the broiler. Leftovers can be used to make a tasty stuffed omelet.

Ingredients :

Two smoked trout, approximately ten inches in length each

- ¼ cup cooking fat (preferably ghee).

Cooking tip: To make the fish even more delicious, sprinkle it with finely chopped chervil, chives, parsley, and tarragon after brushing it with fat in step 2.

Guidelines:

1. Broiler: Preheat to high.

2. Brush the trout with cooking fat to ensure it is well coated. Put it inside the broiler pan.

3. After 4 minutes of broiling, turn the dish halfway through.

4. After transferring, serve warm on a plate.

Snow Crabs

Preparation 5 minutes || Cooking 25 minutes

You can save time by simply reheating and seasoning snow crab legs that are orange-red, which indicates that they have already been cooked. Serve with a side of melted butter or ghee for a delicious dinner.

Ingredients :

- Two pounds of frozen snow crab legs

A tsp of salt and heated water

- Ghee or another preferred cooking fat at room temperature

Guidelines:

1. Fill a pot with enough water to cover the crab legs. Bring the water to a boil and add one teaspoon of salt.

2. Simmer for about eight minutes, or until the crab leg clusters are tender.

3. After removing the legs from the water, gently shake off any remaining moisture.

4. If necessary, add more salt to the meat's garnish. Serve the meat hot, with butter or ghee on the side.

Ten-Minute Skillet Shrimp
Preparation 5 minutes || Cooking 10 minutes

Shrimp adds a tangy and salty flavor that goes well with shredded Parmesan cheese. Shrimp is also easily found and cooks quickly. Every shrimp has a thin coating of cheese on it, which adds a delightful texture to every bite.

Ingredients :

- One pound of medium shrimp, peeled and deveined
- A tablespoon of cooking fat, such as ghee
- A single teaspoon of salt

- Two tablespoons of Parmesan cheese, shredded if desired

Add-ins For Flavor: Serve the shrimp over zucchini noodles, or "zoodles," to make it into a scampi for vegetarian connoisseurs and visitors.

Guidelines:

1. Give the shrimp a good rinse.

2. Melt the cooking fat in a large skillet over medium heat.

3. When the shrimp are fully cooked and pink, add them and stir-fry for about seven minutes.

4. If desired, add cheese, and season with salt. Stir to combine, then serve hot.

Salmon Steaks On Grill
Preparation 10 minutes || Cooking 10 minutes

Take off your shoes, enjoy the sunshine, and inhale the fresh air while you grill outside. You can use any fish that catches your attention, even salmon steaks.

Ingredients :
- Four wild-caught, 1-inch-thick salmon steaks
- ½ cup divided Ghee or another preferred cooking fat

Add-ins To Taste:

Season with salt, garlic powder, and lemon pepper after brushing in step 2. Present alongside grilled asparagus and Portobello mushrooms.

Recipe Advice:

The salmon will pull off the grill by itself when it's done. Check for white beads on the fish's surface and sides to see if it's overcooked.

Guidelines:

1. Assemble the barbecue.

2. Thoroughly coat the salmon steaks with cooking fat.

3. Place the steaks on a well-oiled grill, about 4 inches above the heat source.

4. Using a flat spatula, flip the salmon steaks once they are cooked through, which should take about 6 minutes. Reapply the oil.

5. Continue to grill the steaks for an additional 4 minutes, or until a fork can easily pierce them.

6. Let it rest for five minutes, then serve warm.

Sea Bass Wrapped In Bacon

Preparation 10 minutes || Cooking 30 minutes

This recipe creates a soft, tender white fish covered in crispy bacon strips using the same methods as the popular ketogenic dish, bacon-wrapped scallops.

Ingredients :

- Two tablespoons of grass-fed butter or heritage pork lard
- Four 6-oz fillets of sea bass
- Twelve strips of raw bacon

Guidelines:

1. Warm up the oven to 190°C, or 375°F.

2. Put parchment paper on a rimmed baking sheet.

3. Drizzle the sea bass filets with some of the cooking fat. With the bacon seams down on the sheet, encircle each fillet with three pieces of bacon.

4. Bake for approximately 25 minutes, or until cooked through and flaky. Reheat the meal.

Swordfish Roasted
Preparation 5 minutes || Cooking 20 minutes

This is a family favorite lunch recipe that comes together quickly and needs minimal cleanup, taking less than five minutes to prepare.

Ingredients :

- 2-pound steaks of swordfish
- A solitary teaspoon of salted seaweed
- Two tablespoons of your favorite cooking fat, such as Ghee.

Purchase Advice:

See Mountain Rose Herbs' selection of culinary salts for high-mineral salts.

Guidelines:

1. Set oven temperature to 175°C/350°F.

2. Transfer the fish steaks to a baking dish that is ovenproof. Coat the fish generously with salt and then cover with cooking fat.

3. Bake for 20 minutes, or until the fish reaches your desired doneness. When cooked, a fork should easily be able to flake the fish.

4. After transferring, serve warm on a plate.

Sandwiches With Stuffed Cheese Salmon
Preparation 5 minutes || Cooking 20 minutes

These delicious "sandwiches," which taste like another meat dish, have flavors reminiscent of the ingredients that make up sushi rolls: salmon and cream cheese.

Ingredients:

- 1/4 cup of Country Home Cream Cheese, at room temperature
- Four boneless, thinly sliced salmon fillets
- 1/4 cup ricotta cheese (organic)
- Salt

Enhancement of Flavor:

To the cheese mixture in step 3, add minced onion, garlic, or rosemary (oregano, chives, or rosemary).

Guidelines:

1. Set oven temperature to 175°C/350°F.

2. Put parchment paper on a rimmed baking sheet.

3. Combine the ricotta and cream cheese in a small bowl.

4. Place two salmon fillets on the baking sheet, skin-side down.

5. Evenly divide the cheese mixture between the two fillets.

6. Top with the remaining fillets, skin-side up. Add a little salt to taste.

7. The salmon should be baked for 20 minutes, or until it is cooked through. Reheat the meal.

Surf 'n' Turf
Preparation 5 minutes || Cooking 20 minutes

Add a savory, fatty, and salty flavor to your home cooking that will satisfy your palate and perfectly capture the essence of recipes that are carnivorous in nature.

Ingredients :
– Four 6-oz haddock filets
- One pound of pork ground
- Ghee or Heritage Pork Lard

Add-ins To Taste:
Instead of using ground pork, use sausage (pork, beef, chicken, or bison). Consider

experimenting with alternative ground meats.

Guidelines:

1. Set oven temperature to 400°F, or 204°C.

2. In an ovenproof or cast-iron skillet, cook the pork over medium heat, stirring often to break up any clumps. Bake for about five more minutes, or until well cooked and browned.

3. Evenly distribute the pork throughout the pan. Arrange the haddock filets so they are not touching. Place them on top. Drizzle some cooking fat over the top.

4. Put the object inside the oven. Bake for 12 to 15 minutes, or until the fish pierces easily with a fork. Reheat and proceed to serve.

Baked Trout with Sausage Compound

Preparation 15 minutes || Cooking 1 hour + 5 minutes

A hint of herbal flavoring is common in sausage. If you would rather not taste the herbs, you can use ground pork in place of the sausage. The North American Game Fish Cookbook had the original recipe, which called for homemade sausage. Designed for family-style fishermen, this cookbook was published in the 1970s. I chose to stick to the same formula.

Ingredients :

- Two pounds of whole trout
- A half-pound sausage

Notable Nutrients: Selenium, calcium, magnesium, phosphorus, potassium, sodium, and vitamins A, B3, and B12 are all present in trout. Its fat-to-protein ratio is also 2:1.

Historical Note: Native to North America west of the Rockies are rainbow trout and steelhead. With the exception of Antarctica, they are currently found in practically every state and continent due to their rising popularity.

Guidelines:

1. Set the oven's temperature to 175°C/350°F.

2. If necessary, Take the trout and give it a thorough rinse in cold water.

3. After taking the sausage out of its casing, divide it into two equal pieces. Each portion should be rolled into a long, narrow roll that matches the cavity of the trout in length. Place the sausage rolls inside the fish cavities.

4. Seal the edge of every trout directly over the sausage filling, wrapped in aluminum foil.

5. With the cavity side up, put the trout in a 9 x 13-inch baking pan.

6. After an hour of baking, take off the foil to reveal the sausage.

7. When the sausage is golden brown, place the dish 2 inches under the broiler

and broil it for 5 minutes. After fully removing the foil pouch, serve hot.

Basic Seafood Chowder
Preparation 5 minutes || Cooking 30 minutes

I adore this thick and creamy soup from my childhood memories of eating at an old, rickety seaside house and eating chowder from a bread bowl, even though I now live in the mountains and follow a ketogenic or low-carb diet.

Ingredients :
- Two tablespoons of ghee or other cooking fat
- Clam juice, half a cup
- One clam pound
- A single cup of chicken stock

- One cooked pound of langostinos

- A cup of organic heavy cream for whipping

- A single teaspoon of salt

Guidelines:

1. In a medium saucepan over medium heat, melt the cooking fat.

2. Add the clam juice and broth and stir. Simmer until the liquid reduces, covered, about 15 minutes.

3. Place the clams and langostinos into the pot. Increase the heat, bring to a simmer for ten to fifteen minutes, and then turn it down to a gentle boil.

4. After adding the cream, season with salt. Add five more minutes of simmering. Reheat the meal.

Chapter 8

MUSCLE MEATS RECIPES

Meatballs
Preparation 10 minutes || Cooking 20 minutes

These can be eaten in batches and are delicious and cold as leftovers. For a daring twist, try replacing part of the ground beef with ground beef heart. As you become used to the flavor, start with a 50% ground beef-to-ground beef ratio and adjust.

Ingredients :

- Two pounds of ground beef raised on grass
- A single tablespoon of salt

Add-ins For Flavor: Serve these meatballs made from beef hearts to the whole family. After removing half of the meat, add the chopped cilantro, onion, and garlic. Tailor the seasoning to your dining companions.

Cooking Tip: To make meatballs, use any ground meat (bison, lamb, etc.).

Guidelines:
1. Set oven temperature to 175C/350F.
2. In a bowl, combine the meat and salt.
3. Form 2-ounce balls with the palm of your hand.

4. The meatballs should be baked for 20 minutes in a glass baking dish, such as a Pyrex 9 by 13-inch dish. It's okay if the balls come into contact with one another.
5. After serving warm, chill any leftovers.

Bombs of mozzarella meatballs
Preparation 15 minutes || Cooking 20 minutes

This meat-loving "fat bomb" is far superior to peanut butter cream cheese ones! Experiment with different cheese flavors; blue and brie cheeses make excellent mozzarella substitutes.

Ingredients :

- Eight ounces of whole milk mozzarella cheese that is organic
- One pound of beef ground
- One tablespoon of salt

Cooking Tip: Make double the amount and keep them chilled for a ready-made, super quick meat meal.

Guidelines:

1. Set oven temperature to 175C/350F.

2. In a bowl, mix the meat and salt. Divide the cheese into eight equal parts.

3. Form the meat into 2-ounce balls with the palm of your hand. Using your thumb, create a well in the center of each ball and press a cheese cube into it. Pack the meat into the opening.

4. The meatballs should be baked for 20 minutes in a glass baking dish, such as a Pyrex 9 by 13-inch dish.

5. After serving warm, chill any leftovers. Ideal as chilled leftovers.

Beef Burgers
Preparation 5 minutes || Cooking 10 minutes

There are serious cravings for these greasy, salty, golden brown burger patties, which are aptly named as a carnivore's "fat bomb." Put ice cream and brownies away. When you sandwich two patties together and spread some grass-fed butter in between, you'll be swooning!

Ingredients:
- Two tablespoons of Pioneer Style Tallow
- One pound of ground beef raised on grass

- Salt

Taste Add-ins: Add this recipe to your weekly meal prep and serve it with lettuce wraps or your favorite low-carb bun. Use homemade mayonnaise and fermented pickle relish from The Ketogenic Edge Cookbook as garnish.

Guidelines:
1. Heat the cooking fat in a skillet over high heat.
2. Form burger patties with your hands. Two or four-ounce patties work best for basic macro tracking.
3. After heating the skillet, place the burgers inside and cook for two to four minutes. Turn the food and continue

cooking until the desired doneness is achieved.

Burgers With Cheese Made Of Bison
Preparation 5 minutes || Cooking 10 minutes

To make these, use bison fat if it's available; if not, use butter or Pioneer Style Tallow. Strong cheeses like smoked Gouda, goat cheese, Brie, or raw cheddar pair well together for the optimal flavor profile.

Ingredients:

- One pound of bison meat
- Eight slices (ounce) of organic cheese
- One tablespoon of fat for cooking

- Salt

Add-ins For Taste:

Serve with your favorite toppings, like bacon, avocado, red lettuce, grilled onions, and mushrooms, and you're sure to please the whole family. Kids particularly love grilled pineapple on burgers!

Guidelines:

1. Heat the fat in a skillet over high heat.

2. For easy macro tracking, divide the burger patties into 2- or 4-ounce portions with your hands.

3. Place the burgers in the hot skillet and cook for two to four minutes.

4. Flip each burger over, place a slice of cheese on top, and cover with a lid.

Simmer for a minute or two more, or until the cheese is melted and cooked to your desired consistency.

5. Season generously with sea salt and serve warm (though cold is equally good).

Cheeseburgers With Bacon
Preparation 10 minutes || Cooking 10 minutes

These perfectly cooked, juicy beef burgers with crispy bacon and melted cheese on top are the definition of carnivorous heaven. Every bite has a perfect harmony of meatiness, tanginess, and saltiness. Perfect for breakfast, dinner, or lunch.

Ingredients :

A one-pound portion of grass-fed ground beef

- One teaspoon of salt

- 1 tablespoon of cooking fat or Heritage Pork Lard

- Four ounces of organic cheese each

- Four slices of cooked, uncured bacon

Guidelines:

1. Ground beef and salt should be combined in a big bowl. Shape four quarter-pound burgers.

2. Heat the lard in a large skillet or cast-iron pan over high heat.

3. When the burgers are hot and piping hot, add them to the skillet and cook for 2 to 4 minutes.

4. Flip each burger over, place a slice of cheese on top, and cover with a lid. Simmer for a minute or two more, or until the dish is cooked through and the cheese is melted.

5. Place the patties onto plates, then place a piece of bacon on top of each one.

Pan-seared Chops Of Lamb
Preparation 15 minutes || Cooking 5 minutes

These easy and satisfying lamb chops are a great way to highlight the rich, delicate, and grassy flavor of lamb and are perfect for any night of the week.

Ingredients :
- 1/4 cup of butter or lamb fat melted in the grass
- A single tablespoon of salt
- Eight rib chops of lamb grown on grass

Add-ins To Taste:

Usually accompanied by a mint sauce. Pulse 1 bunch of fresh mint, a cup of fresh parsley, 2 anchovy fillets, and 1 clove of garlic in a food processor. As needed, drizzle in additional olive oil once the sauce has just the right amount of looseness. Adjust the salt to taste.

Guidelines:

1. In a large bowl, mix the salt and fat to make the marinade.

2. Toss the lamb chops in the marinade and let them sit for 10 minutes.

3. Set a heavy-bottomed skillet or cast iron over high heat. For an even brown crust, cook the chops for two to three minutes on each side. A meat thermometer should

read 130. F (55 C) for a medium-rare finish.

4. Give the chops a few minutes to rest on a platter before serving. Season with more salt and fat, if desired.

T-Bones House Steak
Preparation 1 Hour|| Cooking 5 minutes

T-bones, or any steak, are best pan-seared and then finished in the oven. This is a family-favorite recipe. This method produces an exterior that is slightly crusted and browned, with a juicy, tender interior.

Ingredients :

- Two 16-oz, 1-inch-thick, bone-in, grass-fed T-bone steaks
- 4 tablespoons of olive oil for cooking
- Salt

Recipe Advice:

If you are short on time, you can omit the step of letting the steaks come to room temperature, but it does help to ensure more accurate cooking times. To keep them hot before serving, tent or loosely cover with foil after plating in step 5.

Guidelines:

1. Set the oven's temperature to 415. F (212 C) first. Remove steaks from the refrigerator thirty minutes before cooking to allow them to come to room temperature.

2. Season generously on both sides with salt, and let sit for five minutes.

3. Heat an ovenproof skillet to a high temperature and add cooking oil. Once the oil is scorching hot, sear the steaks for up

to two minutes. Turn and sear the other side for a minute more.

4. Put the pan in the oven and bake it for two or three minutes, or until it's medium-rare or rare.

5. Place steaks on a platter and pour the same amount of juice over each one. Let rest for 5 minutes, then serve warm.

Burgers With Broiled Butter
Preparation 5 minutes || Cooking 10 minutes

Though these broiled butter burgers, which are infused with butter from the inside out, offer an alternative preparation technique, ground beef is one of the easiest meats to make.

Ingredients :

- Eight ounces of chilled butter made from grass
- Two pounds of grass-fed ground beef

Recipe Advice:

Use your favorite compound butter flavor in place of butter in step 2.

Guidelines:

1. Heat the broiler first.

2. Form the meat into four half-pound patties.

3. Divide the butter into eight portions of one ounce each. Put four slices of butter aside and place one inside each burger.

4. Burgers should be broiled until desire is achieved.

5. Place the last slice of butter on top of each patty and return it to the broiler until the butter melts and sizzles.

6. Garnish hot servings with salt, if desired.

Melted Cheese And Meatloaf
Preparation 10 minutes || Cooking 10 minutes

My kids will tell you that dinner is quite filling just with cheese. Like content campers, they savor every bite of this cheesy meatloaf.

Ingredients :

- Six big, natural eggs
- One pound of meat or pork minced
- Two ounces of Country Home Cream Cheese, room temperature
- One cup of organic cheese, shredded

Guidelines:

1. Set oven temperature to 175C/350F.

2. Spread some cooking fat in a small loaf pan.

3. In a large bowl, beat the eggs lightly. Mix in the cream cheese after adding the meat.

4. Place the mixture into the pan that has been greased, then bake for 30 minutes.

5. Take it out of the oven, give it a five-minute rest, and then evenly distribute the shredded cheese on top.

6. Put the oven back on and broil the cheese for five minutes, or until it becomes bubbly and golden.

7. Before serving, let it rest for an additional five minutes.

Cooked Goat Leg With Broth
Preparation 5 minutes || Cooking 24 Hours

Since they can live in areas where cows cannot, goats are an excellent choice for people who want to raise animals but have limited space or resources. Goat meat, usually tough and lean, can be softened and made into almost melt-in-your-mouth deliciousness by slow cooking. Savor goat meat for breakfast, covered in butter and sprinkled with sea salt from Cyprus.

Ingredients :

- An optional cup of apple cider vinegar

- A single goat leg

Cooking Tip: Slow cooking is key to getting moist and tender goat meat. To make a large stockpot, ask your butcher to break the joints.

Guidelines:
1. Transfer the goat leg to a large stockpot, add the vinegar (if using), and cover with water.
2. Keep it covered by checking the water level every few hours while simmering on low heat for the entire day.
3. To remove the broth, use a fine-mesh stainless steel strainer or a colander lined with cheesecloth.

4. Accompany the heated meat with a cup of broth and serve.

Tri-Tip Roast
Preparation 1 minutes || Cooking 45 minutes

Usually served as a roast or steak, tri-tip is a delicate and lean cut of bottom sirloin. This time, we're highlighting the roast, which is well-known for its superb flavor and reasonable cost.

Ingredients:
- One roast tri-tip grown on grass
- A tablespoon of finely ground salt
- Cooking fat

Cooking Tip: A meat thermometer reading of 125 F (55 C) is ideal for medium-rare.

Guidelines:

1. After adding salt, cover and chill the tri-tip for the next day.

2. Before cooking, let it come to room temperature for 30 to 45 minutes and then season with salt once more.

3. First, heat a skillet over high heat and preheat the oven to 425. F (218 C). Put in some cooking fat.

4. For three minutes on each side, or until a golden-brown crust forms, sear the tri-tip.

5. Move the contents to a sheet pan equipped with a wire rack and roast for 8

minutes, modifying the cooking duration as necessary.

6. Before serving, let it rest for a minimum of ten minutes. Serve warm, thinly sliced against the grain.

Sirloin

Preparation 5 minutes || Cooking 10 minutes

This is a family favorite that we usually serve with lots of browned butter. Savoring every steak bite as we sit around our little wooden table. To create the ultimate experience, combine plenty of fat with the steak juices.

Ingredients :

- One tablespoon of tallow or butter from grass-fed cows
- Two pounds of 8-ounce top sirloin medallions
- Salt

Cooking Tip: After searing the meat, place the skillet in a preheated oven for one to two minutes to achieve an oven finish akin to Steak House T-Bones.

Guidelines:

1. A big, heavy cast-iron or stainless-steel skillet should be heated to a high temperature.

2. Heat with the addition of cooking fat. When the steaks are hot, sear them for up to two minutes on each side, or until a crust forms that is golden brown. For medium-rare, adjust to 4 to 5 minutes per side.

3. Before serving, allow the meat to rest for a minimum of five minutes. Sprinkle with

salt after making a thin slice against the grain.

Delectable Skirt Steak
Preparation 10 minutes || Cooking 10 minutes

The easiest steak to prepare is the famous skirt steak. It comes from the plate, nestled between the brisket and flank, and its long, flat shape is perfect for fajitas, Chinese stir-fries, and churros. Braising in bone broth or searing will intensify the flavor.

Ingredients :

- A single 2-pound grass-fed skirt steak

One teaspoon of salt

- 1/4 cup of cooking fat or butter from grass-fed cattle

Guidelines:

1. Season the meat with salt and rub it with cooking fat.

2. Put a big frying pan on high heat. Cut the steak in half against the grain if it won't fit lengthwise, and cook it in batches.

3. The steak should be seared for 4 minutes on each side to form a golden-brown crust.

4. At least five minutes should pass before slicing the meat thinly and serving it warm.

Brown Butter Steaks With Ribeye
Preparation 5 minutes || Cooking 10 minutes

Brown butter, just regular butter heated until the milk solids toast, adds a delightful depth and nutty flavor to a premium cut of steak.

Ingredients :

- Four tsp butter from grass-fed cows
- A single tablespoon of salt
- A pair of 8-oz ribeye steaks

Important Nutrients:

Steaks with ribeye are high in essential fats that are vital to overall health. Their

1:1 protein-to-fat ratio makes them the preferred option for many ardent followers of the ketogenic diet.

Guidelines:

1. As directed, season the steak with salt.

2. Heat a skillet over medium heat, then add the butter and gently brown it. Set it aside.

3. Reheat the pan to a high setting.

4. Sear the steaks for about 2 minutes on each side, or until a golden brown crust forms.

5. Melt the butter on top of each steak and serve hot.

Marinate-free Bbq Kebabs
Preparation 50 minutes || Cooking 15 minutes

This recipe works well for grilling chicken, tri-tip roast, thick loin steak, strip steak, or even chicken on hot summer days.

Ingredients:

1/4 cup beef raised on grass
- Four teaspoons of grass-fed butter, or Pioneer Style Tallow
- A single tablespoon of salt

Recipe Advice:

For stability, make sure each kebab has two skewers.

Add chopped onions, mushrooms, and zucchini to a grill to enhance the flavor. Lemon juice, olive oil, minced garlic, dried oregano, basil, salt, and pepper are used to marinate the vegetables.

Guidelines:

1. Give the skewers at least 30 minutes to soak in the water.

2. Cut the meat into cubes that are 2 inches in size, and then skewer it, leaving space between each piece.

3. Coat the meat with cooking fat.

4. Grill both sides for 10 to 15 minutes. Accompany with a side of Creamy Goat Cheese Sauce for dipping.

Steak New York Style
Preparation 15 minutes || Cooking 10 minutes

New York strip steaks are a popular choice at American steakhouses because of their tenderness and strong beef flavor.

Ingredients :

- A single tablespoon of salt
- One pound of steaks from grass-fed strip loin
- 1/2 cup of fat used for cooking

Historical Observation:

The most common term for this type of steak is "strip loin," though it is also known by other names, such as "New York strip steak" and "Kansas City strip steak."

Guidelines:

1. Preheat a skillet by turning the heat to high.

2. Season steaks with salt and/or fat.

3. Sear steaks for about 2 minutes on each side, or until done as desired.

4. When the steaks are five minutes out of the oven, turn them over and serve with the pan juices.

Roasted Chuck
Preparation 40 minutes || Cooking 4 Hours

Cheap and reliable chuck roast is transformed into a flavorful dish with a distinctive sauce by Dutch oven deglazing.

Ingredients :

- One 2-to 3-pound roast of grass-fed beef chuck
- Two tablespoons, divided, of coarse salt
 Four glasses of bone broth
- Cooking fat

Recipe Advice:

If you do not have access to a Dutch oven, use an ovenproof deep pot.

Guidelines:

1. After lightly salting the roast, put it in the fridge to rest for the entire night.

2. Once it's at room temperature, reseason with salt.

3. After searing, put the roast in a hot Dutch oven.

4. To deglaze the Dutch oven, add broth.

5. Put the roast back, cover with half of the liquid, and simmer.

6. Simmer for approximately 4 hours over a stovetop or in an oven preheated to 300F. Before serving, take a fifteen-minute break.

Beef Sirloin Roast

Preparation 20 minutes || Cooking 45 minutes

A top sirloin or strip loin roast is elevated to a new level of flavor when roasted in the oven thanks to Dutch oven deglazing.

Ingredients :

One roast top sirloin or strip loin, two pounds, three to four inches thick
- Four tablespoons of cooking oil
- Salt

Recipe Advice:

Always place the meat on its "fat side" for a moist oven roast.

Guidelines:

1. Preheat the oven to 425 F.
2. Season the roast with salt.

3. In hot cooking fat, brown the roast for three minutes on each side.

4. Bake for about 35 minutes, or until a meat thermometer reads 125 F.

5. After fifteen minutes, turn off the heat, cover, and leave it alone.

6. Garnish with salt and serve warm.

Fillet Mignon: "Better Than The Restaurant"

Preparation 5 minutes || Cooking 10 minutes

Filet mignon's delicate texture and subdued beef flavor make it an opulent dish that's ideal for cooking at home. Cleaning up after this one-pan wonder is a breeze.

Ingredients :

- A pair of 8-oz filet mignon steaks raised on grass
- Olive oil for cooking
- Kosher Salt
- Compound butter, if desired

Guidelines:

1. Set oven temperature to 175C/350F.

2. Warm up a big, heavy skillet on high heat.

3. Apply oil grease to the skillet. The steak should be seared for two minutes on each side, or until a brown crust forms, in a hot skillet.

4. Cook the skillet for three to six minutes in the oven after moving it there. When a meat thermometer reads 125 F (55C), medium-rare, remove.

5. Slice the steak thinly against the grain after letting it rest for at least five minutes. Season with salt and serve warm, garnished if preferred with Compound Butter.

Slow-cooked Stew With Beef

Preparation 5 minutes || Cooking 2 hours + 20 minutes

This dish is a hearty soup with rich bite-sized pieces that melt in your mouth. Collagen and connective tissues from the bones and tail of the beef are abundant in it.

Ingredients :

- Two pounds of bones from grass-fed beef
- Two pounds of stew beef raised on grass
- One 4-pound beef oxtail raised on grass
- Sea salt

- Optional herbs and vegetables

Cooking Tip:

Tougher cuts of beef, like round, sirloin, or chuck, are best prepared slowly.

Guidelines:

1. The marrow bones should be placed in the middle of a slow cooker.

2. Add stew beef on top and oxtail around the outside.

3. Ensure that the bones and meat are completely immersed in water.

4. Reduce heat and simmer for 12 to 24 hours, or until fork-tender.

5. Heat with or without the broth. Meat leftovers can be reheated in butter or

added to other dishes, like omelets. Season with salt, to taste.

Simple Roasted Ribeye

Preparation 15 minutes || Cooking 2 Hours + 30 minutes

A whole-standing ribeye roast is a stunning centerpiece for holiday feasts, offering flavor and beauty in equal measure.

Ingredients :

- A single cup of melted cooking fat
- One 6-pound roast of bone-in ribs
- Sea salt

Cooking Tip:

Generally, one rib should be enough to feed two people, but you can adjust the serving sizes to accommodate different preferences.

Guidelines:

1. Start the oven at 500. F, or 260 C.

2. Using a sharp knife, score the roast and then liberally season with salt and cooking fat rub.

3. Once the fat has been trimmed, transfer the roast to a roasting pan.

4. Roast for thirty minutes, then reduce the heat to 325. F (163 C) and continue cooking for an additional two hours, or until the meat is medium-rare.

5. Take out of the oven, put foil over it, and leave it to rest for fifteen minutes before slicing it and serving it warm. Pour some juice over each piece.

Grilled Shaved Beef
Preparation 15 minutes || Cooking 15 minutes

Shaved steak is a common ingredient in cheesesteak sandwiches and is very easy to prepare, making it the perfect choice for busy kitchen days.

Ingredients:

One pound of shaved steak from grass-fed cattle

- Olive oil for cooking

- Sea salt

Cooking Tip:

Serve with hot Cracklings for even more texture contrast.

Guidelines:

1. Heat a cast-iron pan or skillet.

2. Heat it and add the cooking oil.

3. The steak should be lightly browned after two to three minutes of salt. ing.

4. After allowing it to sit for a minimum of thirty seconds, add some salt and serve it hot.

Seared Flat Iron Steak
Preparation 5 minutes || Cooking 30 minutes

Flat iron steaks, cut from the shoulder, are very flavorful and can be eaten on their own as an appetizer or grilled.

Ingredients:

- Two 8-oz flat iron steaks raised on grass
- One tablespoon of salt, plus extra to taste
- Olive oil for cooking

Cooking Tip:

Try completing the optional overnight seasoning prep steps for optimal results.

Guidelines:

1. Salt the steaks and chill them for the night if you'd like.

2. Before cooking, let the steaks come to room temperature for 30 minutes and then season with salt once more.

3. Over high heat, preheat a heavy skillet or cast-iron pan.

4. Add the fat to the skillet and sear the steaks for two minutes on each side, or until a brown crust forms.

5. After turning off the heat, leave it to rest for five minutes or more, and then thinly slice it against the grain. Season with salt and serve warm.

Round Roasted Eye
Preparation 45 minutes || Cooking 1 Hour + 5 minutes

Serve leftovers with a dollop of chilled Country Home Cream Cheese to balance out the leanness of the roast.

Ingredients :
- One round grass-fed beef roast
- Four tsp finely ground salt
- 4 tablespoons of fat for cooking

Guidelines:
1. Season the roast with salt, then transfer it to a plastic bag and refrigerate overnight.

2. The roast will come to room temperature if it is left out on the counter for 30 to 45 minutes.

3. Set the oven's temperature to high and preheat it to 275. F (135 C).

4. After adding the cooking fat, sear the roast for three to four minutes on each side, or until a crust forms.

5. Transfer the roast to a sheet pan fitted with a wire rack and bake it for 1.5 hours, or until the internal temperature of the meat thermometer reaches 125 F (55 C), which is the medium-rare temperature.

6. After removing it from the oven, let it rest for at least ten minutes. Slice thinly against the grain and serve warm.

Slow-cooked Brisket Of Beef
Preparation 35 minutes || Cooking 8 Hours

Pot-cooked brisket makes an incredibly simple dinner that is fork-tender. When done right, it has a rich flavor and mouthwatering texture that make the wait worthwhile.

Ingredients :

An entire 4-pound grass-fed beef brisket
- Bone broth, two cups

Flavoring Add-ins:

Add aromatics like bay leaves, thyme, onions, and carrots and simmer.

Cooking Tip: Select a flat cut with a top fat cap to keep moisture during cooking.

Guidelines:

1. Pour liquid into a slow cooker until two-thirds full, then add the brisket and broth.

2. Cook on low for 8 hours, or until fork-tender.

3. Give it at least 30 minutes to rest in the juices. The brisket is done when it is easily torn along the edges without breaking apart.

4. Transfer the liquid on top and serve hot. To taste, add salt.

Chapter 9

RAW MEAT ORGANS AND BONES RECIPES

Bone Broth
Preparation 5 minutes || Cooking 24 Hours

To make a nourishing broth, combine meaty bones, knuckle bones, and marrow bones; simmer for an extended period of time. Enjoy it warm in stews, soups, or meat and seafood braising.

Ingredients :

- Four to six pounds of bones from animals fed grass (bison, goats, lambs, etc.)
- One-fourth cup raw apple cider vinegar

Cooking Tip: To improve the flavor of the broth, dry roast the bones in the oven before adding them to the pot.

Savings Tip: After the broth cools, remove the tallow layer to use as cooking fat.

Guidelines:

1. Pour water over the bones in a stockpot or crockpot and mix in the apple cider vinegar.

2. Simmer at a low temperature for at least 18 hours and up to 48 hours. Simmer without boiling, adding water as needed to keep the contents submerged.

3. After cooking, remove any scum that has gotten solid on top.

4. Once the mixture has cooled, strain it through a fine-mesh strainer to remove the meat, marrow, and collagen from the bones.

5. The broth can be refrigerated for up to five days or frozen for an extended shelf life.

Broth With Chicken
Preparation 10 minutes || Cooking 12 to 24 Hours

Chicken broth can be flavored with carrot, onion, garlic, celery, and parsley—a remedy our great-grandmothers used. For the last two hours of cooking, you can add optional ingredients.

Ingredients :

– Ten water cups

A tsp of unrefined apple cider vinegar

The bones of a whole chicken that has been slow-cooked or roasted in the oven.

Notable Nutrients: Add chicken feet to boost collagen, amino acids, and minerals.

Guidelines:

1. Transfer the vinegar and water into a slow cooker or stockpot. Add the chicken, cover, and cook for 12 to 24 hours on low or over low heat. Just keep it simmering; don't bring it to a boil.

2. Remove any excess fat from the broth's surface. Let cool, then strain through a fine-mesh strainer or cheesecloth.

3. Before transferring them to long-term storage containers, freeze in ice cube trays or store in glass jars in the refrigerator. Each ice cube offers tiny portions of convenient thawing.

Liver Dipped In Butter
Preparation 45 minutes || Cooking 5 minutes

Savor the unparalleled taste of butter-crusted sheep liver, a popular recipe that's easier to make than beef liver. Examine your options for liver, including those from pig, lamb, goat, bison, veals, and chickens.

Ingredients :
- 1/4 cup butter made from grass
- One pound of calf or beef liver
- One sheep's liver
- Salt

Cooking Tip: Soak the liver for at least 30 minutes in a thick brine before cooking.

Guidelines:

1. Soak the liver for at least 30 minutes in a thick brine before cooking.

2. Once the outer membrane, any fat, and tubes have been removed, slice the organ into ¼ to ½-inch thick strips.

3. In a skillet or frying pan, preheat the butter over medium heat.

4. To the hot, foamy butter, add the liver. When turning, wait until the edges are firm; cook the second side for 30 to 60 seconds after cooking the first for 60 to 90 seconds.

5. Warm and well salted, serve.

Elevated Meat

Preparation 10–20 Minutes ||
Fermentation Period: 1–3 Months

Taste-tested meats that have undergone fermentation may be some of the most potent foods available. Icelanders have a cultural affinity for hákarl, or fermented shark, while the Inuit ferment a variety of animals for up to a year to produce what Vilhjalmur Stefansson called "highmeat" with euphoric and energizing effects.

Ingredients :

- Any fresh liver or muscle meat

Guidelines:

1. Slice the liver or meat into small pieces
or slivers.

2. Transfer the meat halfway into a jar.

3. To allow oxygen to enter and to stir the
contents for greater surface area exposure,
keep the jar refrigerated and open it two or
three times a week.

4. After one to three months, it is ready to
eat, and the longer it is kept unopened, the
better.

Carpaccio
Preparation 10 minutes || Chill time 1 Hour

Carpaccio, an appetizer-style Italian dish of raw meat or fish, is made with thinly sliced or pounded meat. This technique yields a tasty meal and works well with a range of meats.

Ingredients :

- Eight ounces of grass-fed beef tenderloin

Guidelines:

1. The meat should be frozen for an hour or until it solidifies.

2. Slice the meat thinly into 1/8- to ¼-inch pieces after removing the wrapper. Till the slices are paper-thin, gently pound them between sheets of butcher paper.

3. Divide the meat among chilled plates and serve cold.

Caviar à la Louche
Preparation 5 minutes || Cooking 0 minutes

The roe of wild sturgeon fish is traditionally referred to as "caviar". On the other hand, it is more commonly used to incorporate fish roe from various species. This delicious treat, which is high in omega-3 fatty acids, DHA, EPA, vitamins D and B12, and trace minerals, can be served simply for a delicious dinner.

Ingredients :

- A quart of caviare

Guidelines:

1. From the jar that is open, take a spoonful of caviar.

2. Consume it uncooked or incorporate it into fancy recipes like Boiled Eggs or Buttery Baked Cod.

Burgers With Liver
Preparation 5 minutes || Cooking 5 minutes

Leftover ground beef burgers, crispy fried eggs, and soft liver combine to create a tasty and simple lunch or breakfast. Add it a slice of pungent cheese, like smoked Gouda or Danbo, for an added burst of flavor.

Ingredients :

- Two hamburger patties per day
- Four to six pieces of baked liver with butter
- Two teaspoons of fat for cooking
- A pair of free-range, organic eggs

Guidelines:

1. Burger patties and liver should be warmed again and then put aside.

2. In the skillet with cooking fat, fry the eggs.

3. Put an egg on top of each burger patty.

4. Serve the hot egg on a plate with the liver covering it.

Bits Of Gelatin

Preparation 10 minutes || Cooking 4 Hours

Snackle up with Gelatin Bites and Carnivore Jello for a clever way to fend off hunger. Without adding a lot of calories, gelatin soothes the lining of your stomach and gives you a slight feeling of fullness. You can change the flavor by adding things like vanilla extract, nutmeg, and ground cinnamon.

Ingredients :

- Water
- Four teaspoons of grass-fed beef gelatin

Guidelines:

1. Pour a cup of water into an 8 by 8-inch glass baking dish.

2. Spread the gelatin evenly over the surface of the water and allow it to bloom for ten minutes.

3. Two cups of water should be placed on the stove.

4. Stir thoroughly after adding hot water to the gelatin.

5. Once firm, refrigerate for approximately four hours, and then cut into small pieces.

6. Store the jello bites in an airtight container at room temperature.

Hearts Of Beef Meatballs

Preparation 10 minutes || Cooking 20 minutes

I usually include meatballs in my weekly menu, and this recipe is perfect for those who love organ meat. Organ meats can be introduced with ground beef and beef heart mixtures in different ratios, such as 50/50 at first and then gradually working your way up to 25/75. You can try meatballs made entirely of beef heart later.

Ingredients:

Ground beef heart, one pound

Guidelines:

1. Set oven temperature to 175°C/350°F.

2. Form two-ounce meatballs with your hand.

3. Transfer them to a glass 8 x 8-inch baking dish.

4. After 20 minutes of baking, let cool and serve warm.

Pate Beef Liver
Preparation 20 minutes || Cooking Overnight + 5 Minutes

Liver can be hard for people who are not used to eating organ meats. A great place to start is with a creamy pate made from liver that has been fed grass. It tastes good on its own or combined with ground heart crunchies or bacon strips.

Ingredients :

- 1/4 cup beef liver raised on grass
- Half a cup of butter from pasture
- One-half cup unrefined heavy cream
- Salt

Guidelines:

1. Follow the Guidelines in the butter-bathed liver recipe to prepare the liver.

2. After letting it cool slightly, puree it with butter, cream, pan drippings, and salt in a food processor.

3. The mixture should be chilled for at least five hours or overnight in glass ramekins or other containers.

4. Present it chilled.

Liver Pate Chicken
Preparation Overnight+ 5 minutes || Cooking 5 minutes

A good substitute for beef liver if you're not a fan of the taste is chicken liver. It tastes good, is inexpensive, and can be found in big quantities, either fresh or frozen. A tasty substitute is this blended chicken liver pate, sautéed in butter from grass-fed cattle.

Ingredients :

One-pound trimmed livers of chicken

- 1/4 cup butter made from grass

- Salt

- One hard-boiled egg (may be skipped).

Guidelines:

1. Melt the butter in a skillet and cook the livers until browned and well done.

2. Blend them with pan drippings and season with salt once they've cooled.

3. If desired, you can add a hard-boiled egg and process it once more until it's smooth.

4. Pour the mixture onto a plate, cover and chill for the entire night, then serve chilled.

Pemmican
Preparation 5 minutes || Cooking 0 minutes

Dried and finely ground meat, heart, and liver are combined with salt and Pioneer Style Tallow in the Native American preservation process known as pemmican. It's very nourishing and portable, which makes it perfect for camping and hiking. You can experiment with different meats and organs using this recipe.

Ingredients:

- Seven ounces (200 grams) of dried, ground meat

- 5 oz (150 g) of dried heart, ground finely

- 2 oz (50 g) of dried liver, finely chopped

- Two teaspoons of salt

- Pioneer Style Tallow, 16 oz/450 g

Guidelines:

1. Heat the tallow until it melts.

2. In a bowl, mix meat powder and salt.

3. Melted tallow should be completely covered over the dried meat mixture and well mixed.

4. Roll the pemmican into squares, balls, or molds.

5. After letting it cool, store it in an airtight container away from the sun.

Delicious Beef Heart Meats

Preparation 10 minutes || Cooking 15 minutes

Ground beef and beef heart combine to create a flavor that is well-known, mild, and has more nutrients. Organ meat lovers will love this recipe; if they'd rather, they can use ground beef heart only. For a tasty twist, add extra cheese on top.

Ingredients :

- One pound of ground beef
- One tablespoon of grass-fed butter or cooking fat
- Ground beef heart, half a pound
- Salt
- Two free-range, organic eggs
- 1/4 cup of raw milk cheese, shredded (optional)

Guidelines:

1. Set oven temperature to 400°F, or 204°C.

2. In a skillet with butter, brown the meat and season with salt.

3. After beating, mix the eggs with the meat.

4. Spoon mixture into glass pie plate; sprinkle optional cheese on top.

5. Allow it to rest for five minutes after baking for fifteen to twenty minutes, then reheat.

Crispy Liver
Preparation 10 minutes || Cooking 4-8 Hours

Instead of slicing the liver, you could ask your butcher to grind it for you. Spread out the liver on a dehydrator tray after it has been ground. Then you can dip these unusual chips into Carnivore Crab Dip, Creamy Goat Cheese Sauce, or Beef or Chicken Liver Pate.

Ingredients :
- Liver fed on grass (any animal)
- Optional: Sea salt

Guidelines:

1. Slice the liver into thin strips, then spread them out flat on a dehydrator tray. If you'd like, you can season with salt.

2. The top surface should continue to dry on the "meat" setting until it feels totally dry. Continue drying after flipping until the food is completely crunchy. As an alternative, you can bake on a sheet at 155°F (70°C) until they are dry.

3. Store it in an airtight container.

Pasta Lamb Testicle
Preparation 5 minutes || Cooking 15 minutes

I'm not sure why I included this recipe, but maybe you'll be intrigued enough to give it a try. Grilling brings out the best flavor and adds a touch of smoke to the gamey gland. The outer membrane crisps and chars, but the inside meat stays juicy. Testicles are often likened to scallops in texture.

Ingredients :

- A single lamb testicles pair
- Salt
- Optional: Compound or butter butter

Guidelines:

1. Assemble the barbecue.

2. Season the testicles with salt and grill for ten to fifteen minutes, until the outsides are nicely charred. The tissue might burst as a result of the procedure.

3. Slice into ½-inch rounds and serve hot. If desired, add butter.

Tongue: "Better Than Roast Beef"
Preparation 10 minutes || Cooking 3 Hours

Similar to a pot roast, slow-cooked tongue yields flavorful, tender meat that is devoid of bones and gristle. Once cooked, it is impossible to distinguish between muscle and tongue when the meat is sliced. Cold leftovers are great the next day!

Ingredients :

- One tongue of beef fed grass
- Add as much seasoning as desired (one bay leaf, two garlic cloves, one small Spanish onion, six black peppercorns, and two chopped celery ribs).

Guidelines:

1. After rinsing the tongue, simmer it in a stockpot with optional seasonings for two to three hours, or until it is easily pierced.

2. Peel off the outer layer after letting it cool in ice water.

3. Cut into pieces, serve warm with sauce, or refrigerate to use at a later time.

Uncooked Organ Meats
Preparation 5 minutes || Cooking 0 minutes

Pick fresh, organic organs that have been raised on grass or pasture whenever possible. Combine raw organs with cooked foods to incorporate them into your diet. Try brain with bacon or crispy pork belly, a big marrow spread on an Everyday Beef Burger, or a Bison Cheeseburger with minced liver.

Liver

1. Clean, chop into cubes or thin slices, and eat. Avoid dense arteries and connective tissues.

2. Cut the tip into thin rounds, wash, and consume the heart. Before pan-frying, trim off any excess fat and remove any thick gristle.

3. Divide the material into four sections and trim to fit once you've reached the chambers.

Guidelines:

1. Clean, cut out any pieces of bone, and peel the membrane if you'd like. Cut into pieces or eat whole.

2. Grab the bone, force the marrow out, and eat. If very firm, cut with a knife.

Tartare Of Beef
Preparation 10 minutes || Cooking 10 minutes

This classic bistro dish is simple to prepare at home. A lovely dish that incorporates essential nutrients from our diet is raw beef tartare. Choose lean cuts such as tenderloin, top sirloin, or sirloin for a flavorful meal.

Ingredients :

- Four ounces of steak, lean
- Salt
- One yolk from an egg

Guidelines:

1. After rinsing, pat the steak dry. If you'd like, heavily salt everything and refrigerate for an hour.

2. Take out any tendons or fat from the meat.

3. Cut the meat into cubes and finely mince it with a sharp knife.

4. Season with salt, to taste.

5. Using the minced meat, create an indentation in the center of the plate. Add the yolk as well. For shaping, you may choose to use a cookie cutter.

Grilled Rognons
Preparation 10 minutes || Cooking 10 minutes

The French term for "grilled kidneys" is "rogons grillés." While fresh kidneys from lambs are preferred, kidneys from fresh beef, veal, pork, or other healthy animals also work well. The Ingredients and directions are as follows:

Ingredients :
- Four kidneys
- Lard or melted butter
- Salt
- Compound butter or fats infused with flavor, optional

Guidelines:

1. Get the grill ready.

2. Split each kidney lengthwise without separating the halves, then skin and trim the organs.

3. To keep the kidneys flat, skewer through the ends of each one.

4. Sear on the cut side first over high heat until sealed, then brush with melted fat and season with salt. Cook for 5 to 7 minutes, reducing heat and turning several times until done.

5. Serve hot, with the option to top each kidney with a pat of butter or fat.

Crunchies With Ground Heart
Preparation 5 minutes || Cooking 6-8 Hours

Heart crunchies can be used like croutons and are surprisingly oily. You can sprinkle them over scrambled eggs with cheese fries or serve them alongside bison cheeseburgers. The Ingredients and directions are as follows:

Ingredients :

- One pound or more of ground heart, such as bison, beef, etc.

Guidelines:

1. Using the "meat" setting, evenly distribute the material onto a dehydrator sheet and let it dry. Alternately, bake at 155°F (70°C) on a baking sheet until they are dry.

2. When the top feels completely dry, flip it over and keep going until all of the moisture is gone.

3. Split into fragments and preserve in a sealed container.

Organ Meat Quiche
Preparation 15 minutes || Cooking 15 minutes

These twelve nutritious, simple-to-make muffins are ideal for breakfast. You can have easy access to these amazing cups anytime you need them by doubling the batch. The Ingredients and directions are as follows:

Ingredients :

- Half a pound of ground beef
- Ground beef heart, ½ pound
- Ground beef liver, ½ pound
- Cooking fat
- Three organic free-range eggs

- Salt

Guidelines:

1. Set oven temperature to 175°C/350°F.

2. Over medium heat, lightly brown the meat in the fat.

3. In a mixing bowl, mix together all the ingredients. Add salt to taste.

4. Pour evenly into a muffin pan that holds 12 cups.

5. Bake the egg for 12 to 15 minutes, or until set.

6. Take off the heat, let cool for five minutes, and then serve hot. Savor cold leftovers.

Chapter 10

WHEN TO MODIFY OR TRANSIT FROM CARNIVORE DIET

The carnivore diet has become popular due to the potential health benefits of eating only animal products. However, as with any dietary approach, it is important to listen to your body and make adjustments as necessary. In some situations, moving away from the carnivore diet may be necessary.

Many people initially adopt a carnivorous diet to address health concerns, increase energy levels, or explore the potential benefits of a meat-based diet. While some may experience positive results, it is important to be aware of warning signs of change or transition.

Here are six things to consider:

1. Nutrient Deficiencies: A long-term carnivore diet may lead to nutrient deficiencies due to the lack of dietary variety. While animal products do contain essential nutrients, it is important to check blood levels and address any deficiencies with the assistance of a healthcare provider.

2. Digestive Issues: Strictly following a carnivorous diet may cause digestive issues such as constipation or discomfort. Adding low-carbohydrate vegetables or taking fiber supplements may help alleviate these problems. Long-term sustainability depends on paying attention to your body's reactions and making necessary adjustments.

3. Long-Term Sustainability: The carnivorous diet is often a temporary measure. For social, cultural, or personal reasons, some individuals may find it challenging to adhere to the diet for an extended period. A shift towards a more balanced approach that incorporates a variety of nutrient-dense foods can

provide long-term sustainability without compromising health.

4. Athletic Performance: The limited availability of carbohydrates for energy in the carnivore diet may hinder athletic performance for individuals engaging in strenuous physical activities. Targeted carbohydrate consumption during exercise can enhance athletic performance without significantly deviating from the carnivore paradigm.

5. Hormonal Imbalances: The impact of a carnivorous diet on hormone levels varies from person to person. If there are indications of hormonal imbalances, such as irregular menstrual cycles or

fluctuations in energy levels, it is crucial to consult a healthcare provider to address the underlying cause and implement any necessary dietary changes.

6. Weight Management Goals: While the carnivore diet may assist some individuals in losing weight, others may find it difficult to achieve their goals. In these cases, adjusting the diet to include a balanced combination of carbohydrates, fats, and proteins specific to the individual's needs can promote long-term and successful weight management.

The decision to change or abandon a carnivorous diet is a personal one. Making informed decisions about your dietary approach requires regular health checkups, paying attention to your body's signals, and consulting medical professionals or nutritionists. Ultimately, the primary goal for long-term well-being should be a sustainable, balanced diet that meets each individual's unique needs in terms of health and lifestyle.

How You Incorporate Other Food For Balanced Diet

Diversifying food choices is crucial in achieving a balanced diet that takes into account individual preferences and health goals, while also ensuring adequate intake of essential nutrients.

Here are some tips for incorporating a variety of foods in your diet:

1. Fruits and Vegetables: Include a variety of colorful fruits and vegetables in your meals. You can eat them raw or cooked in different ways like smoothies, fruit salads, stir-fries, and salads.

2. Whole Legumes and Grains: Incorporate complex carbohydrates, fiber, and protein by adding legumes like lentils, chickpeas, and beans, and whole grains like quinoa, brown rice, and oats to your diet.

3. Nutritious Fats: Use healthy fats from avocados, nuts, seeds, and olive oil to add flavor and essential fatty acids to your meals. You can add them to your diet in various ways like avocado toast, nut butter on whole-grain bread, mixed nuts as snacks, and drizzling olive oil over salads and vegetables.

4. Dairy Products and Substitutes: For calcium, protein, and other essential nutrients, include dairy products like

yogurt, cheese, and milk in your diet. If you're lactose intolerant, go for substitutes like almond milk, coconut yogurt, and tofu-based cheese. These foods can be eaten on their own or combined with other foods to make smoothies, desserts, or used in baking and cooking.

5. Non-Meat Sources of Protein: Meat is the primary source of protein, but other plant-based substitutes like tofu, tempeh, seitan, and dairy products can be incorporated in your diet to increase nutrient diversity and liveliness of meals.

6. Spices, Herbs, and Dressings: Add flavor to your meals with herbs, spices, and

condiments like mustard, salsa, and vinegar. They make your meals more interesting and satisfying without adding significant calories or macronutrients.

7. Drink plenty of water: Keep yourself hydrated by drinking water throughout the day. You can also include unsweetened beverages, herbal teas, and fruit, herb, or cucumber infusions to add flavor without calorie or sugar additions.

8. Consuming With Mind: Eating mindfully is essential to improve the dining experience and promote a positive relationship with food. Savor the food's flavors, chew slowly, and take your time

during meals. Be aware of cues indicating when you are full or hungry.

Incorporating a range of foods in your diet provides enjoyment, satisfaction, balance, and support for overall health. You can make your meals more interesting and satisfying by experimenting with different ingredients, flavors, and cooking techniques. Consult a registered dietitian or nutritionist for tailored advice and suggestions based on your specific dietary needs and goals. Remember, moderation and balance are the cornerstones of a sustainable and healthful eating pattern.

Chapter 11

COMMON CHALLENGES AND SOLUTIONS

It can be difficult to navigate typical obstacles to leading a balanced lifestyle, but with perseverance and resilience, one can get over these obstacles. I've recognized some common issues and offered workable solutions to successfully address them based on my observations and personal experiences.

1. Time Restrictions:

Making time for exercise and meal preparation is frequently a challenge when juggling work, family, and personal obligations. But it's crucial to put self-care first. Weekend meal prep, making non-negotiable fitness appointments, and outsourcing work when practical are some solutions.

2. Emotional Eating and Cravings:

Emotional triggers have the potential to cause unhealthy food cravings, which can undermine efforts to maintain a balanced diet. Journaling and deep breathing are two mindfulness exercises that can assist in recognizing emotional cues. Exercises that refocus attention and reduce cravings include yoga, meditation, and walks.

Social Coercion:

3. It can be difficult to navigate social gatherings where unhealthy food is abundant. But dialogue is essential. Providing friends and family with information about dietary preferences and restrictions promotes understanding and support. Bringing a dish to share also guarantees that options are in line with individual health objectives.

4. Insufficient Drive:

It can be difficult to stay motivated to keep up healthy habits when faced with challenges and setbacks. Motivation can be rekindled by establishing reasonable objectives, acknowledging minor accomplishments, and surrounding oneself with encouraging people. Recalling the "why" behind starting the journey can be a very motivating thing.

5. Economic Limitations:

People are frequently discouraged from making healthy changes because they believe that living a healthy lifestyle is costly. However, eating healthily can be made affordable by setting financial priorities, shopping wisely, and choosing whole, seasonal foods. You can also save money by looking into free or inexpensive exercise options, like working out at home or outdoors.

6. Insufficient Awareness:

It can be intimidating to navigate the vast landscape of fitness and nutrition information. Consulting with credible authorities, like certified fitness professionals or registered dietitians, can yield precise and customized guidance. People who take the time to learn and try new things are better equipped to make decisions.

7. Progress on Plateauing:

Reaching fitness or weight loss plateaus can be demoralizing. Plateau periods, however, are normal and present chances for introspection and modification. Rekindling progress can involve reviewing objectives, adjusting schedules, and adding fresh challenges, like attempting a novel exercise routine or attempting new foods.

8. Perfectionism and Self-Criticism:

Burnout and self-criticism are frequent results of aiming for perfection. A positive outlook is fostered by accepting self-compassion and expressing gratitude for any accomplishment, no matter how tiny. Perseverance and resilience are fostered when obstacles are reframed as chances for development.

9. Insufficient Help:

Starting a health journey alone, without a network of support, can be lonely. On the other hand, asking for help from like-minded people, whether in person or online, develops a sense of accountability and community. Participating in online forums, group activities, or fitness classes promotes encouragement and connection.

10. Impractical Anticipations:

Excessive ambition in goal setting can lead to disappointment. Long-term success is instead encouraged by prioritizing progress and sustainable changes over perfection. Honoring progress milestones promotes sustained development and strengthens virtuous behaviors.

On the road to a balanced lifestyle, one must overcome typical obstacles with persistence, patience, and a proactive attitude. People can overcome obstacles and ultimately reach their health and wellness objectives by embracing setbacks as learning opportunities and putting workable solutions in place. Recall that progress is a process rather than a destination, and that every accomplishment, no matter how tiny, is cause for celebration.

Conclusion

ADDRESSING COMMON INQUIRIES

1. Question: Can I eat vegetables on a carnivorous diet?

Reply:Vegetables are generally not allowed on a carnivore diet because it is based on animal products. However, some people choose to include a small amount of low-carb vegetables.

2. Question: Do I need to eat organ meats on a carnivorous diet?

- Reply: While organ meats are optional, they are nutrient-dense and provide important vitamins and minerals that can improve the overall nutrient profile of the diet.

3. Question: Can I have dairy on the carnivore diet?

- Reply: Some people strictly follow an animal-only diet, while others include dairy products such as butter and cheese. Whether or not to include dairy depends on personal goals and tolerance.

4. Question: How can I get enough fiber on a carnivorous diet?

- Reply: Carnivorous diets naturally lack fiber, so people may need to take supplements or eat low-carb vegetables to support digestive health.

5. Question: Can I have tea or coffee on a carnivorous diet?

- Reply: Black coffee and unsweetened tea are generally allowed on a carnivore diet, but individual preferences may vary.

6. Question: Is the carnivorous diet appropriate for athletes?

- Reply: While athletes can follow a carnivorous diet, they may need to adjust their macronutrient intake to maintain optimal performance. Finding the right balance requires experimentation.

7. Question: How do I manage social situations on a carnivorous diet?

- Reply: Letting friends and family know about your dietary choices and bringing your own carnivore-friendly dish to events can help ensure appropriate options are available.

8. Question: Can I drink alcohol on a carnivorous diet?
- Reply: While alcohol is generally avoided on a carnivore diet, some people may choose to consume dry wines or spirits occasionally. It's important to be aware of possible effects on tolerance and ketosis.

9. Question: Does the carnivorous diet cause digestive problems?
- Reply: Digestive changes may occur initially as the body adjusts to the new

diet, but they usually improve over time. Drinking enough water and reducing fat intake can help.

10. Question: How do I deal with cravings for non-carnivorous foods on a carnivorous diet?
- Reply: Overcoming cravings can be facilitated by staying committed to the diet, experimenting with different meat cuts, and finding filling substitutes.

11. Question: Can I follow a carnivorous diet if I already have health issues?
- Reply: It's important to consult a healthcare professional before starting any restrictive diet, especially if you have

underlying medical conditions. They can provide personalized advice.

12. Question: How does a carnivorous diet affect cholesterol levels?
- Reply: The effect of a carnivorous diet on cholesterol levels can vary depending on the individual. Regular monitoring and professional advice are recommended.

13. Question: How can I prevent nutritional deficiencies on a carnivorous diet?
- Reply: Eating a variety of meats, including organ meats if desired, and getting routine blood testing and expert advice can help prevent nutrient deficiencies.

14. Question: Is fasting recommended on a carnivorous diet?

- Reply: Intermittent fasting is sometimes combined with a carnivorous diet, but it's a personal decision that may depend on individual preferences and goals.

15. Question: Can I follow a carnivorous diet while pregnant or breastfeeding?

- Reply: Pregnant or nursing women should consult medical professionals before implementing any restrictive diet to ensure optimal nutrition for both mother and child.

16. Question: How does a carnivorous diet affect gut health?

- Reply: A carnivorous diet can have different effects on gut health. While some may experience changes initially, others may report improvements. Consuming fermented foods or probiotics can support gut health.

17. Question: Can a carnivorous diet lead to muscle growth?
- Reply: A carnivorous diet, along with resistance training, can help gain muscle. Adequate protein intake is necessary for muscle development.

18. Question: Can I use spices and condiments on a carnivorous diet?
- Reply: Spices and salt are commonly used on a carnivore diet. Depending on

personal preferences, plant-based ingredients or condiments without added sugar may also be used.

19. Question: How does a carnivorous diet affect energy levels?

- Reply: Energy levels may fluctuate initially as the body adjusts to the new diet, but maintaining adequate fat intake, electrolyte intake, and hydration can help support consistent energy levels.

20. Question: Can I have cheat days on a carnivorous diet?

- Reply: Whether or not to have cheat days is a personal choice.

9 798880 185795